Choose Health for your Children

LaDean Griffin

Copyright © 2000 by LaDean Griffin

First Printing: 2015

DEDICATION

To my husband Bob
and our children

Connie
Wally
Mark
Lynn
Cindy
Scott

Whom I love more
than words can say.

PREFACE

It was said quite prophetically by Brigham Young in his Journal of Discourses, 15, page 225:

"Would you want doctors? Yes, to set bones. We should want a good surgeon for that, or to cut off a limb. But do you want doctors? For not much of anything else, let me tell you, only the traditions of the people lead them to think so: and here is a growing evil in our midst. It will be so in a little time that not a woman in all Israel will dare to have a baby unless she can have a doctor by her. I will tell you what to do, you ladies, when you find you are due to have an increase, go off into some country where you cannot call for a doctor, and see if you can keep it. I guess you will have it, and I guess it will be all right too."

His prophecy became the case when I was having my babies. The first three of my children were born the hard way with doctors and drugs. By the time I became pregnant with my fourth child. Natural childbirth was becoming popular, but not without a doctor. Some doctors were beginning to try the method. My younger sister had three children the natural way with no pain. So when she heard I was pregnant she sent me the book, Childbirth without fear, by Grantly Dick Read.

Having read the book, I became convinced enough to try it. I found a young new doctor willingly to help me with a no anesthetic, natural childbirth. I began Mr. Read's recommended exercises faithfully. I lived on the things I understood personally using nothing but fruits, nuts, vitamins, minerals, etc. I practiced the positive affirmations each night before I went to sleep.

I would say over and over to myself "there is going to be no fear and no pain in having this baby. I will have this baby in the morning when I am rested."

About the time I was almost ready to deliver, I found an un-stamped letter in my mailbox from my young doctor. Who had become afraid to deliver a baby the natural way and informed me to find another doctor. I found an older doctor who seemed interested in what I was trying to do, and said he would take my case. One morning I awoke with beginning labor and called the doctor. I then proceeded to take my own enema before leaving the house.

We arrived at the hospital and were seated in the waiting room to wait for labor to proceed. While waiting I practiced my breathing exercises and felt very comfortable. In a short time the doctor came in and took me to the delivery room. I asked him not to chain me to the table as was the usual procedure and he agreed. Soon a nurse tied something to my wrist that I could use as an anesthetic. I kept pushing it away and she asked if I wasn't in great pain. And I said no. Finally the doctor said to her, "Leave her alone she want's to do this herself."

The baby girl was born at 8:10 in the morning when I was rested. There was no pain and no bleeding. What a wonderful way to have a baby. Later on in that evening, a nurse came and asked me if I was going to nurse my baby. And when I said yes she said, "You will want some coffee or milk then." I said, "No I don't drink coffee, and I don't drink milk. Could you please bring me some fruit juice?" She said, "You can't nurse your baby without milk." And I said, "cows don't drink milk to make milk they eat grass." And she went out and slammed the door.

The method to have a baby the natural way, except for the diet, is better said and taught by Grantly Dick Read. His book can usually be found in the library. There are also other books available since his book was written. But his teaches easily a wonderful truth.

There are many amazing wonderful truths to be found in the following pages. There are things that parents need to know in order to bless the lives of their children. May you find these truths and how to apply them to reduce pain and suffering is my sincere hope.

LaDean Griffin

TABLE OF CONTENTS

CHAPTER 1

HUMAN NEEDS

At the request of my husband and some of my children, I pick up my pen to write about the care and feeding of babies and children. My father, J. Melvin Gibby, said;

"The greatest legacy you can leave to your children is
a strong, clean body,
a wholesome, alert, and truth seeking mind,
a listening ear,
a clear eye,
a level head,
a love of mankind,
a desire to serve,
a will to achieve,
an honest and prayerful heart,
an unshakeable faith in God,
a desire and determination to keep his commandments,
and the memory of your own righteous example as a guide."

I came from a father and mother who loved their children deeply and were thankful to be parents and set a wonderful example for each of their children. Even during the depression, my father and mother worked very hard to provide us with the necessities of life, physically, emotionally, intellectually, socially, and spiritually.

Each human that enters this world has these same five basic needs, whether he is born in the most remote place on the earth or in a so-called civilized city. I would like to address each of these needs.

MENTAL AND EMOTIONAL

Man is a reasoning being who must learn to make correct computations and come to rational conclusions in order to achieve success. He has a great need to accomplish and succeed, and through such accomplishments, he can make himself comfortable.

The first experiences begin the process of learning, as each feeling in the newborn's life makes an impression on the brain. All new experiences have to attach to another, like a tree growing and branching out. If the child is healthy and the brain is well, learning and developing proceeds rapidly. This is the reason it is so important for the mother and father to understand that they are creating a body, sick or healthy, with which they will be associated, day in and day out, until the child is grown. The child will not only be subject to its mother's whims during pregnancy, but it will reflect the love and care of its parents from the day of its first breath.

Is the mother well-developed and happy to welcome the child with love, or does she reject the child as a bother? The parent figure can be a poor example, lazy, or selfish, and too self-centered to take care of the child's needs, or perhaps lacking in the financial necessities for proper food, etc. Then there are parents who are just plain mean. There is also the loving parent who is thankful to have the child.

Just as the mental environment is an important factor in a child's development, his emotional attitude is subject to the kind of care he is receiving. Is there love and parental support to learning, or no motivation influence? It is a well-known fact that the child who is loved, played with, cuddled, and talked to, learns much faster than the child who is neglected in these areas. If any of the needs of the baby are not met, a mental stress begins in the brain, which is similar to panic, and causes a distrust of the adults around the child, a disruption in its mental, as well as its physical development, and possibly even a fear for its life.

In the time frame of the computer age in which we live, more and better opportunities have developed, if parents are willing to take advantage of them. Even if parents are uninterested in teaching their child, a child can learn more, just from television or by accident than a child could a few years   ago. There was no way we could develop computers without realizing the importance of the computer that each man, woman, and child carries on his shoulders.

A few years ago, the idea emerged to teach people that if they wanted a better life, they had to think positively. Religion had been teaching, since time began, to have faith. Now however, in the age we live in, a computer and correct programming is a tangible, undisputable fact. If you want your computer to be true in its information, you must give it the correct data.

Thinking men and women have become more analytical and are demanding correct answers. Seekers after truth of the laws of the universe, find the truth, and as the wealth of knowledge spews forth in all kinds of literature and world media - from pornography to scripture - the books are open to all manners of choices in learning. It almost appears you can get to heaven or hell faster than a decade ago. There are even books on how to teach a baby to read, and books on how to toilet train a child in four or five hours.

PHYSICAL

Physical is always closely associated with mental. If the body is sickly, enthusiasm for life and leaning are greatly impaired. Mans body was intended to go and do. Man struggles with the continuing desire to be free from pain. From a tiny baby, he learns what pain is and how to avoid it with his limited knowledge. As you watch a baby overcome the most difficult obstacles, from crawling, walking or climbing up into a chair, you observe that when he once reaches his goal, he has to go back and do it over and over again, no matter how difficult it was. He often proves to himself and others that the pain he suffers is worth the final result. Babies show great courage and curiosity and a lust for learning which is often lost in adults. If the child is fed poor food, filled with poison spray and chemicals, drugs, or if he has birth defects, his courageous job of learning how to go and do is greatly hampered. Often a mother may have good intentions, but incorrect information; therefore, she places a stumbling block in her child's way unknowingly. Then, when he gets sick, she takes him to the doctor who administers drugs and adds insult to injury. The physical development is also involved with an inborn need to express and receive love, which will eventually result in the need to create new life. A child has a need to be comfortable. All humans have a need to be comfortable. All that a baby can do to ask someone to make them comfortable is to cry. It makes absolutely no sense to spank a child who is asking for help. A wise mother will discover what the need is and will fill that need.

One of the most important things necessary for a happy, well-adjusted baby who learns rapidly is a schedule that the baby can depend on. Too often the baby's schedule interferes with selfish wants of parents, so his schedule is haphazard. A sleeping schedule is as important as an eating schedule. A child who is properly fed, and develops good sleeping habits will be a happy child. Somehow people learn to train their dogs, but do not realize that a child must also be trained from day one. A dog trainer would never hit his dog with his hand. He would use a newspaper. The punishment of striking a child with the hand will only create hate. Hands should be used to love and reward, not to punish.

SOCIAL

Man is a social being with a need to belong and be loved and respected. He needs the approval first of his parents, then of society. He needs high self esteem. He cannot tolerate rejection. He needs to be able to communicate. A child needs to be loved enough that he is taught to behave properly in a social setting. He must learn from the beginning that he is being taught manners so that other people will like him and he will be accepted in his society. Some parents arrive at the mistaken idea that everyone will think their little darling is cute and funny no matter how badly he behaves. It is not true parental love that allows a child to be a law unto himself, at an early age. It is destructive and unfair to the child. How can he belong if he is obnoxious and uncaring about those around him? He must learn that all of the negative traits are unacceptable behavior. That includes everything from screaming to get his own way, meanness, lying, cheating, hatred, stealing, or whatever evolves in a child's life who is undisciplined and untrained.

When there is so much lack of communication in the world today, so much divorce because of social maladjustments, it would appear that more concern for the child's social behavior is necessary to make for happier adults.

The child needs to know that there are rules and laws, both physical and spiritual and that he or she has to abide by rules. If the parent is not consistent in teaching this principle and helping the child create the habit of obedience to laws, the child will generally make up its own mind and develop habits of being contrary and demanding to have its own way. In doing so, the child cannot have all the positive needs met that will result in happiness.

Whenever my children misbehaved in public, I said to them, AI will always love you no matter how naughty you are, but other people won't necessarily love you or even like being around you unless you behave. And I want other people to like you."

A mother's love for her child should be like the pure love of Christ, an unconditional love. A child has to be able to make mistakes in order to learn. As he corrects his mistakes, he needs great approval. If he does not correct them, he needs to know someone still cares and will always strive to help him overcome his problems.

The key to helping the child develop socially is being consistent so the child always knows where you stand on every issue. I never spanked my children because they always knew what I expected of them. In reality, the child wants to please you, his parent. And he has to know what will please or displease you so you must be consistent in your actions toward him so he will know how to act.

SPIRITUAL

Man has a need for some hope in someone other than man. He has an inborn need to worship. He needs peace of mind in a world where everything and everyone eventually dies. If he is secure in the knowledge of the existence of God, he has greater courage or less fear to contend with as his relationship with God becomes his own and not his parents, he will have even greater peace of mind.

Relationships with the things of the spirit are always based on the principles of righteousness. One's ability to obey the social rules of God makes for a happier life seasoned with kindness, love, giving, caring, trusting, helpfulness, and being in control of emotions such as fear, anger, hate, sexual appetites, etc. When a person is in this type of life style, a spiritual closeness to God makes their life even sweeter.

Spirituality is not something one can teach a child by any other means than to teach them the rules and set a good example. There are many social negatives which can be overlooked where the punishment from other people is concerned and the punishment from God seems remote and somewhere far off in the distance, no matter how they have been taught. Then again, some may have been taught well and when they are out from under parental control, are fascinated with the risk of evil. The scriptures tell us, "Teach a child when it is young, and when it is old, it will not depart from it." Sometimes it takes until the child is old for him to realize that he has always been fighting against truth and the path he has chosen in the long run, was the way of pain and sorrow.

Principles of honesty and good manners are often easier to learn than the weightier principles of the laws of God. What the child who rebels against such laws does not understand is that man is that he might have joy and in order to have joy he must have God in his life, and in order to have God in his life, he must live a worthy life. Not that God will not love him but he cannot bless him. He misses so much in his life not to have the companionship of God to help direct his paths. Then on the other hand, how long would a parent take continual abuse from a child? How long will God be abused, before punishment will be given? The scriptures tell us that God will not always strive with man. How long can a person be a law unto himself? Hence a child cannot be forced to obey the laws of God when he is grown. Man has his free agency, and if he chooses hell instead of heaven, that is his choice. If he chooses evil rather than good, society will punish him as well as God, but that is still his choice. That is what life is all about - do we want evil or good. The universe has very definite rules, and one is given the opportunity to make the choice.

When a child is young, the choices are made for him and hopefully they are good for his proper development. The sooner the child becomes a responsible person, the sooner the parent can trust him to be on his own and do the right thing. A parent would not give a baby a butcher knife to play with; neither would the parent let a child drive a car until he is properly trained. Training in all facets of a child's life makes a great difference in the child's confidence and self esteem, provided the child is continually learning obedience to the laws of the world by that which he suffers. The parental role is one of the most difficult jobs in the world, and can be one of the most hurtful or the most wonderful. In order to give a child all four major foundations in their life development, of what I call the four pillars of his temple, the parent must be continually concerned with each pillar. There never can be complete happiness without full maintenance of each of these pillars. A person's temple could not stand if one or more pillars is underdeveloped.

CHAPTER 2

HOW THE BODY FUNCTIONS AND HEALS

After more than 50 years of observation relative to cleaning the body and watching people heal themselves with fasting and sem-fasting methods, I am amazed that it has taken so long for the trend regarding the protein theory to be reversed. The conclusion that protein does not build the body has been long overdue. Today it appears, however, that anyone who is in step with the times or has any real knowledge at all about good nutrition has decided that a high protein diet is passe'.

It is interesting to note that most of the speakers for the National Naturopathic Convention held in San Francisco in 1981 were PhD scientists. Science itself appears to be ahead of medical science with the latest health discoveries.

Dr. Linus Pauling was far ahead of his time. But people like Dr. Linus Pauling or anyone else who wanted to study food or vitamins had a difficult time finding funding.

The hospitals and medical schools have also been supported by the drug industry which holds a tight reign on maintaining only drug use in their education. Most available monies for research were slanted more toward drug research than food, vitamins, or herbal studies. When I read through the volumes of scientific medical research papers that dealt with trivia and came to no helpful conclusions, I wondered how the people could have been fooled for so long.

Let us define mild food (fruits and vegetables) and see why this is the basis of all healing. Fruits are digested in twenty - thirty minutes because they are glucose, a simple sugar. Vegetables, however, digest within forty-five to sixty minutes, when not mixed with concentrated foods such as starch, meat, and complex sugars. Concentrated foods cause the body to work harder and for a longer period of time in the process of digestion, requiring from four to six hours. Pork requires nine hours.

When any of the organic body functions are impaired in any way, the body accumulates waste more readily and eliminates it with greater difficulty. Mild foods are more easily digested and moved out of the body, sweeping debris with them in the process (since both fruits and vegetables, especially those high in ascorbic acid are effective in dissolving mucus), while the bulk acts like a broom. This is much like the action of a detergent on an engine to clean it: the debris and mucus has become chronically lodged itself; then the natural oils of the vegetables and fruits found in the skins and seeds and roughage act similarly to the additive molybdenum disulfide used in engines to reduce the friction and cause longer life of the engine. It has been popular for this reason to use a soft polyunsaturated oil to help move cholesterol from the blood, for cholesterol is nothing more than mucus waste. The natural oils provide a finer lubricating fluid for all internal organs since they do not become hardened or lodge themselves as do the harder oils found in meat, eggs and hydrogenated or cooked oils. Fruit and nut oils will also become hardened and lodge along artery walls when cooked. Nuts or oil-producing fruit and vegetables, skins of apples, etc., harden when cooked, and are better eaten raw. For less friction and a more natural lubrication of the body organs, raw fruits, vegetables, nuts and soft raw oils should be used. Less labor to digest and change is required in order for them to be utilized, especially in a sick body already fatigued by debris and toxic waste accumulated over years of eating too many concentrated, constipating foods.

It is also logical to use mild food in case of chronic or acute illness, since an adequate amount of hormones, hydrochloric acid, and enzymes are required to bring the concentrated foods into a state where they can be used by the body during this four to six-hour process of digestion.

Most people who are chronically sick do not have an adequate hormone balance so as to accurately make this change, there is then an increase in the toxic waste by virtue of the unutilized foods. Fruit and honey are already glucose sugar and do not need much change. Vegetables have a small amount of starch but still do not require as much body effort in the process of digestion. They also have a cleansing and lubricating action, making them a suitable food for building as well as cleansing, with a minimum of strain on body organs.

There are five main types of foods to be removed from the diet of the sick, in order for healing to take place. We will call them concentrated or mucus-forming foods. As long as any of these foods are being taken into the body, chronic waste will not be eliminated unless it reaches such a state of waste as to destroy the life; then, at this state, nature will force an elimination: a cold, flu, or any acute disease. During this forced elimination, nature does not dig too deeply into chronic disease; she will only take off enough waste to allow life to go on.

In order to clean the body to immaculate and beautiful health, eating mild foods and herbs or fasting are the only ways. As soon as you start on mild food and herbs, you will prove this to yourself. The body will start to eliminate mucus and waste from all avenues of escape. Your nose will drain if chronic disease is in the head area. As your body begins to clear, you will begin to have good and bad days. If your vitality (or your ability to eliminate) is high, you will immediately feel as though you were acutely ill. These bad days only last a short time, as nature only removes a little at a time. Then you will have some good days for a while and you will feel wonderful on those days, often the way you felt at your best in youth. The world will look new, younger and bright as hope for renewal of health begins to strengthen your body.

Then the bad days will return again as nature digs deeper into the body to root our chronic disease. After a few days, the good days return and give you rest as well as hope. As the bad days become further and further apart, you will know you are healing. If vitality is low, you will feel better at first until the elimination starts, sometimes taking as long as three weeks. As this wonderful process happens to you, you will hardly be able to remember how badly you felt when you began your program, so when you have a bad day, it will be a great annoyance.

An acute illness is any illness that puts you in bed: weakness, dizziness, headache, cold, fever, or virus disease. In defining acute illness, let me give you a completely new concept. A cold is nature's way of saving your life. We will call it a nature-forced elimination. When you begin to understand this, you will no longer fear disease. You will realize that nature is in the process of saving your life. So the next time you have a cold, enjoy it and remember you had it coming, you earned it. Let nature do her work, such a marvelous work; and you can help her as you learn the rules.

Not recognizing what bacteria feeds upon, science has explained it as a necessary outcome of conditions with life on this planet, the one form of life must live on another so as to keep a balance of all life on earth, an epidemic being a disaster to man but a triumphant victory for the virus. They talk of resistance to disease but do not really understand what true resistance is. To build an immunity by inoculation has been major study but is not the correct answer. Bacteria, parasites, and microbes do not live on sound healthy tissue but rather upon waste. Bacteria are not the cause of disease, but rather the result.

God did not place us here to be battered about by all manner of germs, to take our chances. When we learn the rules upon which our bodies were created and learn to live by them, real health will make its appearance and will be an amazement and wonder.

Chronic disease is as the dictionary defines it: lasting a long time, also recurring, habits that resist all efforts to eradicate them, fixedness, deep-seated aversion to change and is not easily uprooted nor changed. Whatever name it may be called by, there is really only one disease - it is waste lodged in different areas of the body. The only way chronic disease waste will eliminate is by stopping the intake of highly concentrated foods, or fasting. The reason why medical science is not able to relieve the intense suffering or chronic disease is because they do not understand what it is, much less how to loosen it from its permanent residence.

As your body begins to eliminate the waste, cleansing itself on a mild food diet, you can begin to fast periodically on short 24-hour fast. In the beginning, you should eat more vegetables than fruits; then, as you feel increasingly better, you can begin to eat more fruit, as fruit draws and loosens the waste too rapidly for anyone with serious chronic disease. Fruit is the builder, cleanser, healer and most perfect food for man. Vegetables slow down the process of eliminations somewhat, and concentrated foods bring it to a screeching halt. While your body is cleansing, if you eat the concentrated foods, you will stop the process of elimination.

Even though fruit seems to be the perfect food for man, a fruit diet or a long fast can destroy the body in extreme chronic illness because too much waste moves into the blood stream too fast and reacts as if a poison had been taken. The waste of long standing is literally a poison and too much in the blood at one time can kill the body. Herbs and mild food may be used without concern in the most chronic illness. The body will heal rapidly using only mild food. I have seen this happen time and time again. The body will heal using various herbs and an average diet. I have also seen this. But the combination of herbs, vitamins, minerals and mild food is an unbeatable combination.

Listed now will be the foods I regard as mild foods:

MILD FOOD FOR CHRONIC SICKNESS
All fruits and vegetables (as much raw as possible)
Fruit juice (canned, raw, or frozen)
Vegetable juice (raw only)
Soft oil (raw, cold-pressed)
All nuts (must be raw)
Honey (raw)
Sprouts (alfalfa, bean, grains)
All starch vegetables must be baked at 500 degrees
Potato, squash, parsnips, yams

NO CONCENTRATED FOODS WHEN SICK
Grain
Sugar
Dairy Products
Butter
Eggs
Dried Legumes
Meat
Peanuts
Chips, ECT

When grain and beans are sprouted, nature changes them from a starch to a glucose sugar vegetable. The chronically ill generally do not have the powers of correct hormone balance to change the heavy starch in their own bodies. If nature can make the change ahead of time, before they enter the body, they can become a perfect fuel.

When milk products are place in the sick adult body, they only add mucus. The protein requirements for man are definitely proven by the changes occurring in the milk of the mother at different stages in the development of the child. The amount of protein in the milk diminishes as the child grows older. Starting at 2.38 percent protein at birth, it diminishes to 1.07 percent protein by six months of age.

Cow's milk is 16 percent protein. This could explain the crib deaths from bottle-fed babies: suffocation caused by ingesting too much protein. Babies have an enzyme, gastric lipase, which digests fat in the stomach. This lasts about three years.

In an adult, the liver bile digests the fat; with the heavy mucus building from high protein diets, most adults only compound the problems the liver already has to cope with by adding milk products to their diets. When there are problems with the powers of digestion, as in hormone imbalances, milk can become an added burden and food for the microbe resulting in diseases such as tumors and cancers.

Let me explain how milk can be used, or the dried grains (much, bread, etc.) In a fasting cleanse, say during a famine. If it is used as:
1 glass of milk a day only, or
1 bowl of mush a day only, or
1 slice of bread a day only

Along with sprouted grain to give the necessary Vitamin C, the body will start its process of elimination, because it is now living in a semi-fasting state.

You may choose the mild food as a cleansing diet, or you may want to use the above concentrated foods in the given amounts.

The following will tell you what happens during a healing crisis versus a disease crisis. As you begin to clean your body, you may, after about three months, experience a healing crisis. You will learn that a healing crisis is brought on by obedience to the rules of cleansing the body and that a disease crisis comes as a result of disobedience to the laws of good health. The only way the body will heal is through fasting, semi-fasting, or forced elimination. There is no other way.

HEALING CRISIS

1. Happens only as the body is naturally cleansed through fasting and/or semi-fasting and correct body building foods.

2. Happens only when the body has enough vitality to stand the shock. Anything such as tumors and polyps that are near a body opening will flush out during a healing crisis.
3. Happens when a person feels at their best. You will have said to someone that day, "I haven't felt this well in a long time."
4. Usually takes about three months of correct eating to bring about a healing crisis.
5. Only lasts two or three days at the most. No need to take enema or help in any way, except to stop eating.
6. When the body does not have enough vitality even from correcting and staying on a semi-fasting diet, no healing crisis will occur. Rather, the body will pick off the solid wastes a little at a time and gradually cleanse by sloughing the waste off into the blood stream. The body will continue having good and bad days as the healing process continues. As the bad days are further and further apart, the person will feel increasingly better.

DISEASE CRISIS

1. Happens when the body is too full of mucus and clogged to the limit, as in pneumonia etc.
2. Happens when enough germs are multiplying.
3. Happens when body strength and vitality are lowest.
4. Happens to save the life. If clogging continues at the rate it is going, the person would die because of injury to body organs: poisons in the blood, pumped through the heart, crowding vital organs, as in cancer, etc.
5. Lasts several weeks.
6. Happens sometimes when the body becomes extremely cold, causing the body to squeeze like a sponge, starting an elimination, forcing waste into the blood stream. You do not catch a cold by being cold; you earn it because of what you eat.

Fruits
1. Loosen waste
2. Sustain the body

3. Cleanse

Vegetables
1. Slow down process of elimination somewhat
2. Sustain the body
3. Cleanse

Protein Tests
(When a protein test is given while living on mild food)

A. If results are low
    1. Not enough live food
    2. Not enough herbs to move waste
    3. Obstructions

B. If results are normal
    1. Waste is moving out normally.
    2. Sufficient raw food and herbs are being taken.

Concentrated Foods

1. Do not loosen waste as do fruits.
2. Sustain the body.
3. Cleanse (only in semi-fasting proportions)
    1 glass milk daily, or
    1 sandwich daily, or
    1 bowl of wheat daily, etc.
4. Stop the process of elimination somewhat
5. Sustain when taken in normal amounts and with correct food combination.
6. When taken in excessive amounts:
    Clog the system
    Create mucus and pus
    Chronic disease
    Create food for parasites and germs

(When parasites and germs have enough mucus to feed on, they multiply. When they have grown enough, nature forces an elimination to save our lives.)

When you experience semi-fasting or a mild food diet and watch in your own body the miracle happen, you find the fear of disease as well as the aches and pains leaving your being. What kind of fuel do we really need for the best results, for optimum health, performance, and long life? We tend to place in our stomachs whatever is at hand or is pleasing to the palate and in whatever mixtures, never giving thought as to how this is all combining or to what form of gas and poison the combination may be producing, not to mention what that particular poison may be doing to our body. More research into the types of fuel necessary for human health will be next on the agenda.

OLD IDEAS AND NEW TRENDS

In my books and lectures, I have always claimed that the accepted approach to protein could not be correct because when people with terminal disease stop the intake of meat protein, starch and sugar, they more often than not become well again.

The trend in the past few decades has been advancing toward more vegetarianism, and somehow the people who begin to live in such a way because of ill health or for whatever reason seems to be immovable in their determination to stay on their diet and continue to claim that they feel better.

What about this controversy? Reflecting on some English history of the problem, theory along with recent research from England and the United States may open a view to the complexity of the questions being asked today.

Voit in 1866 had made many measurements to analyze food intake. He concluded man should have:
118 grams protein daily
56 grams fat daily
500 grams carbohydrates daily

At least 3, 055 calories.

PROTEIN

Atwoter believed if a man worked at hard manual labor, he should have as many as 8,000 calories a day. Rubner and Atwoter expanded on Voit's theory, increasing Voit's recommendations.

However, vegetarians were not in agreement with this theory. The diets advocated by these men were high in protein probably because diets in general at that period of time were so high in bread consumption. About the turn of the century, Siven questioned the need for so much protein because he personally had lived on only 30 grams daily of protein while maintaining a 2,712 calorie intake.

Then a man named Chittenden who lived on 1,600 calories a day with 37 grams of protein persuaded the academic athletic world to reduce their protein intake. With this lower amount, it was discovered that athletic efficiency and strength were not reduced. Many even suggested that too much protein would be injurious to the kidneys. This lowering of protein requirement became accepted as normal.

For the first thirty years of the 20th century, new studies were introduced, many base on the family unit.

Widdowson began an investigative program having to do with age. While calculating the amount of food consumed by adults and children with similar characteristic and age, he discovered that there was a wide use of protein. This approach seemed to negate the theory that everyone had to have large amounts of protein in order to stay well.

Occasionally, governments or groups of people decide they need to make statements for the good of the people regarding what they should eat to stay well. They then form committees of experts, usually at the taxpayer's expense, and proceed to solve the problem. Sooner or later, they come out with a pronouncement of recommended allowances.

The U.S. National Academy of Sciences has made many such pronouncements and changed many. The British Medical Association in 1950, The Ministry of Health in London in 1964, the British Department of Health and many others have issued statements concerning protein allowances.

The figures even differ widely between countries on protein allowance, for example in Russia and the European countries. The variation between Britain and the U.S. on ascorbic acid, calcium and iron lead us to believe that any stated allowance must only be an educated guess.

The Department of Health in Britain published a chart in 1973 showing research of protein intake of various nature groups showing the variations in different geographical and ethnic groups and came to the conclusion that 10% of intake should be protein (43 grams for men and 38 grams for women). The British Medical Association's recommendation was slightly higher - 11% recommended.

U.S. PROTEIN CHANGES

The National Academy of Science recommends 0.8 grams of protein per kilogram of body weight, approximately .56 grams for men with an average of 2,800 caloric intake.

U.S. recommended daily allowances are:

Men 11-56 years	44 - 56 grams
Women 11-56 years	44 - 46 grams

As vegetarianism has become very popular in the last few decades, many of the great athletes are turning to meatless diets and maintaining strength and endurance.

Is there some reason for this change to a steady lowering of standard recommendations until in many cases people feel they can live completely without meat? It is true that terminally ill people are resorting to a meatless diet or low protein and getting better. Since people seem to get all the so-called essential nutrients by luck rather than by expert guidance, the theory of a well-rounded diet would seem to be the answer and yet what about all the cancer and heart problems so prevalent today? Many cancer producing elements are being found in a well-balance diet. Have we learned all we need to know about protein? Are there certain proteins we need? Is there a difference between meat and vegetable protein?

Nathan Pritikin (U.S.), with his documented studies, claims our heart trouble and many other diseases are caused from too much oil in the American diet as we try to live on high protein foods. He would lead us to believe that there is too much oil in meat for the amount of protein we get from it. The U.S. Department of Agriculture Handbook # 8 tells us beef has 33% fat and 66% protein. In his lectures, Pritikin notes that developed nations use 40-50% fat in their diet and underdeveloped nations use 10-15% fat. His experiments would appear to be very convincing, and his low protein diets seem to be producing some very interesting results. Where patients have artery closure, meat is excluded 6-12 months at a time on his program.

Is meat and oil the only answer to terminal disease, or are there a few more necessary things that we should learn?

DUTCH AND AMERICAN PROTEIN RESEARCH

During the past decade in developing countries, interest in diet has centered around protein, and until recently, it has been assumed that Kwashiorkor (starvation disease) was caused by a lack of protein.

This concept has been raised in the 70's and the popular attitude world wide (with the exception of the U.S.) is, that as long as there is enough good food to supply energy, the protein needs will take care of themselves.

For so many years, people have been led to believe (especially in the U.S.) that the amount of protein one consumed was the building material of the body and it did not occur to many that there could be a possibility that too much protein might be detrimental. Many books and articles today not only discard the protein theory but suggest that animal protein could have certain metabolic side-effects.

Different countries and ethnic groups have varying recommended amounts of protein. For example, in the Netherlands, some research went as high as 100 protein grams a day, but then found it best to have only 11-12% of the energy derived from protein.

PROTEIN AND CALCIUM METABOLISM

There has been so much research done on protein to determine the amount we should take into our bodies and the studies have not reached any agreement.

A high protein intake in humans heightens calcium secretions in the urine which leads to a negative calcium balance.

In testing the protein consumption of animals relative to their calcium absorption, results have shown that the opposite is true. The larger the protein intake, the more thoroughly the calcium was used by the animal.

Realistically, we can't use the results of animal testings to determine the need of protein in humans. Could it be possible that we have spent millions of dollars doing experiments on many animals, for millions of dollars, which are really unrelated to humans? It is erroneous for us to assume that the result of testing on animals is pertinent to people. For example, the human colon is longer than the colons in carnivorous animals and more conducive to the digestion of fruits and vegetables.

Vegetables and fruits sweep any toxic wastes that may be in the body out quickly - acting like a broom. Vegetables and fruits are processed more readily than meat and starch. There are plenty of sources of protein in the vegetable and fruit kingdoms which don't conflict with the absorption of calcium.

When we add meat to the diet, the process of elimination is slowed down causing the body to retain waste for longer periods of time. Then the food putrefies in the bowel causing gases that poison the body and poisons from the waste in the bowel absorb into the blood stream through the colon wall. These poisons cause many of the diseases that man has become subject to. The smell of the stool is extremely offensive when a person lives on meat. The odor of the gas becomes extremely offensive also. A person living on a mild food diet (fruits and vegetables) after their body has become clean, has no bad stool or gas odor. This should prove something I should think.

A cat has a very short colon and it processes and eliminates its food quickly. Let us recall the odor of the litter box. A cat would live exclusively on meat (mice) if it could.

The scriptures have taught us that, during the Millennium, there will be no killing - the lamb and the lion will lie down together. The lion will eat grass. People won't eat the lamb either. We're also taught that, during the Millennium, man will live to be the age of a tree. How old is a tree? I've seen trees that are hundreds of years old. There is an olive tree in the Garden of Gethsemane in Jerusalem that is 2,000 years old. Brigham Young said that when a man lives to the age of a tree, his food will be fruit.

PROTEIN AND OSTEOPOROSIS

In Western countries, the often occurring bone porousness is now causing a revolutionary hypothesis that large quantities of animal protein causing calcium losses must be compensated by metabolism of calcium from the skeleton. Tests conducted on elderly people in Surinam (a country on the North-East coast of South America ruled by the Netherlands from 167-1975 and know as Dutch Guiana) whose ages were known, showed lower incidences of osteoporotic conditions than among Caucasians.

PROTEIN AND SERUM CHOLESTEROL

Tests done in the 1950's on serum cholesterol caused a general trend that low protein consumption by rats, chickens and monkeys caused a higher cholesterol count. The test, however, did not recognize that a greater number of fats and oils were added to compensate for the low protein.

Recently, however, the nature of protein has been studied and researched by many groups, among them Carroll and Hermus, Terpstra, and Dallinga. Their observations and experimental data showed that there is a relationship between animal protein and arteriosclerosis. It appears that in countries where atherosclerosis and hyper cholesterol are not prevalent, the nutrition is mostly vegetarian.

Still other researcher (Sirtori and Co.) A decreasing effect of type II hypocholesterolism when the diet consisted of little fat and large amounts of polyunsaturated and by using soy protein instead of animal protein. It was also found, using soy proteins, that it caused a slight decrease in serum cholesterol.

It was found that serum cholesterol was lower among Seventh-Day Adventists and people on macrobiotic diets (rice) as compared to meat eaters.

BLOOD PRESSURE

Based on epidemic data, researchers have found that in the developing countries (when protein is from a vegetable origin) that, generally, the blood pressure is lower than in Western Europe. Observations of communes on the North American continent who are on a macrobiotic diet showed blood pressure to be lower, giving them further reason for their assumptions.

Information taken from 210 persons ages 16-29 showed that when more meat was added to their menu, their blood pressure increased. Old ideas and traditions die hard.

INDIA RESEARCH

You may not be getting full benefit from your calcium supplement or the milk you drink because you are mixing your milk or calcium with a high oxalic acid food or drink like grapes, grape juice, or spinach.

When I was a child, I remember my mother making tomato soup and how the tomatoes and milk would curdle until she added soda, which probably neutralized the oxalic acid, allowing it to become smooth and creamy.

An interesting study from India caught my attention regarding the mixing of certain oxalic acid plants with calcium causing the calcium to be unavailable to the body. Oxalic acid is an organic acid found in many vegetables and fruits and other plants in the oxalic and Rumex plant families. Oxalic acid can also be found as produced in the human body. It is found in rhubarb, sweet potatoes, grapes and spinach and some 500 different kinds of oxalic plants. The Indian research was done by Urmila Pringle and B.V. Ramasastri of the Indian Council of Medical Research, Hyderabab, India in 1978.

Statements had been made by Srivastava and Krishnan (1959) and Sengh et. al. (1969) that oxalates could render calcium unavailable to the body but no scientific proof had been offered until the Pringle, Ramasastri experiments were accepted by the British Journal of Nutrition, 40:591 1978.

The effects of water soluble oxalate in Amaranthus leaves which contain high amounts of oxalates were tested with milk. Milk used in the experiments contained 600 mg. Calcium. It was discovered that cooking the Amaranthus leaves and throwing away the water, there was a 90% loss of oxalic acid content of water soluble oxalates originally present in raw leaves. There was no loss of insoluble oxalates. However, the loss of water soluble vitamins such as riboflavin, folic acid and ascorbic acid which were also thrown away in the water was considerable, ranging from 86% to 94%. Minerals F and P were also lost to a significant extent in this cooking process. The F mineral loss was approximately 45% and the P mineral loss being 50%. Beta Carotene, which is the fat soluble vitamin, showed no loss nor did the calcium in the leaves themselves, probably because the calcium is in the soluble form in the oxalate plant.

With this knowledge, it might be well to be aware of taking mixtures of supplements or calcium foods with oxalic foods resulting in the destruction of calcium.

For those of you who like herbs, it might be well to note that most kinds of oxalic plants are grown from bulbs or tubers and have showy flowers in various colors. The leaves and flowers close up for the night. Oxalic plants are often grown in hanging baskets. Wood sorel is an oxalic plant that grows in the woods of North America. Some kinds of oxalic plants can be used in salads and some in South America have roots that can be eaten.

In early studies, spinach and rhubarb were considered to be a cause of kidney stones when cooked. This new study would seem to dispute this theory. If too much oxalic acid is a cause of kidney stones, cooking it and throwing away the water seems to remove most of the oxalic acid, according to this Indian study.

In light of these studies, it would not be wise to take your calcium supplement with tomato or grape juice.

CHAPTER 3
PRENATAL AND NATURAL CHILDBIRTH

Giving birth is one of the most magnificent experiences a woman can have. She becomes one with God in the creation of a new life. All of her finest, most noble attributes come into play.

Prenatal and post-natal care can consist of a number of things that could occur. Listed below are some home remedies to make some of these problems easier without drugs.

NAUSEA

Peppermint tea
Alfalfa mint tea
Where nervousness is the cause;
    Catnip tea
    Hops tea
    Red Clover tea
B complex and calcium gluconate added to the diet helps the nervous system

In Pregnancy:
Goldenseal Root
Calcium gluconate used as an antacid

BLADDER INFECTION

Enema with small syringe and laxative herbs in small amounts
Slippery Elm, approx. 2 tsp. Daily
Goldenseal Root, approx. 3 tsp. Daily
Alfalfa mint tea, approx. 1 cup every hour
Stop eating during infection
Use fruit or fruit juice only
Goldenseal Root will usually stop the bleeding of the bladder with one application.

KIDNEY INFECTION

Enema with small syringe
1,000 mg. Vitamin C every hour
Goldenseal Root, 2 tsp. Daily
Juniper oil or Juniper, in severe cases
Potassium gluconate, 99 mg tablets, approx. 3, twice daily to take off fluid

Kidney Herbs:
Cornsilk tea
Goldenseal Root tea
Juniper Berry tea

Dandelion tea
Alfalfa tea
Sassafras tea
All of the above teas available are diuretic by nature

SYMPTOMS OF LACK OF SULPHUR

If any of these symptoms appear, a deficiency of sulphur is the major cause.

Toxic condition (help elimination)
Disc trouble
Dull hair
Joint troubles
Joyless appearance

Difficulty in talking and singing
Menstruation delayed
Menstruation irregular
Moodiness
Sores do not heal
Voice box gives out easily
Toxemia is not totally the lack of sulphur, but is caused generally
  from a poor diet of long standing.

If the mother to be is under too much stress, she will tend to have more nausea if she is too full of mucus waste, or has low blood sugar, or any nervous condition. When low blood sugar is the cause, the mother does not produce adequate amounts of B6 in the colon, which can cause nausea. Licorice root will alleviate the blood sugar levels and act like the adrenal cortin hormone she cannot produce, much like a diabetic taking insulin. Acidophilus or B6 will help the digestive process by providing the B6 she is not producing.

Any brown skin discoloration on the face (pregnancy mask), hands or arms is an indication that the adrenals are under stress. The glands are unable to produce enough cortin hormones to maintain a correct balance.

The two major hormones produced by the adrenal glands are, cortin, which allows a person to withstand daily stress and worry, and adrenalin, which allows a person to fight or run in an emergency.

The least stressful foods are fruits and vegetables. When a person has any weakness in any of the glands of the body, they build toxic waste faster and eliminate it with greater difficulty than other people whose glands function normally. Therefore, it is logical that they should live on foods such as fruits and vegetables which are less heavy and not mucus forming.

NURSING

Lots of fruit for mother

When a baby has a cold, mother can take up to 1,000 mg. of vitamin C hourly, stay on fruit, and take a laxative. The cleansing of the mother will also purify her milk and heal the baby's cold.

Caked breast can be helped by hot and cold packs. Be sure to empty the breast each time baby is nursed, if possible.

Attention needs to be paid to nipples, washing them during pregnancy, using a soft brush to toughen them, in preparation for nursing, especially for a first baby. When the baby begins to nurse, the nipples can become so sore they will crack and bleed. This is one of the primary reasons that women do not continue to nurse. It has been my experience that none of the so-called nursing ointments work very well. Begin the first day of nursing by putting B.F.I. antiseptic powder mixed with pure lanolin on the nipples in between each nursing. You can mix it yourself or ask the pharmacist to mix it for you. Nipples must be washed before each feeding. Strict attention must be paid to nursing habits if successful long term feeding is to continue.

Nursing should start immediately after birth to give the baby a fluid that will clean out its bowel as well as be a comfort to the child.

When milk comes in, on the third day, if the mother is healthy, she may fill up so full as to leak heavily for several days. This leakage is another reason for sore breasts. A heavy cream such as lanolin will keep the nipples dry underneath, while the B.F.I. powder is an antiseptic that will keep any bacteria from building. This is such a simple procedure, but may make the difference in whether or not you are successful in nursing your baby. If B.F.I powder and lanolin are not available, Vaseline and powdered goldenseal root can be mixed and used. Wash nipples thoroughly with warm water before each nursing.

Strict attention must also be taken to alternate breasts each feeding. If the breasts are bursting with milk and the baby cannot take it all, do not try to empty the breast. Just nurse on the other side the next time. The amount will then regulate to the baby's needs.

If one breast is left past the next feeding and the same breast is nursed again, the unused breast can become caked and very painful. It can even cause fever and the mother can become very ill.

If more milk is needed to satisfy the baby's needs, make sure each breast is emptied at a feeding. It is a good idea to put a safety pin on the bra strap to indicate the last breast emptied or the next one to be nursed, whatever you decide. So often, nursing mothers do not wake up thoroughly enough the way bottle baby mothers do because they do not have to get up and heat a bottle; therefore, nursing mothers may not remember which side she fed the baby on last. Simply forgetting is the main cause of caked breast.

The mother should lay down if possible to nurse her baby, and rest and enjoy her child. In a quiet moment, she cannot only give food to her baby, but also love, comfort, peace, and happiness. Even a mother with many children can give those wonderful moments to the new little one. It can be a sweet and precious time for both mother and baby.

She should talk to the baby, pat it, and cuddle it. As the child grows bigger, it can become a fun time of teaching, playing, smiling, laughing, and loving. There is a closeness that few bottle fed babies ever experience, unless the mother takes those feeding times with her baby. Too often, the bottle fed baby is left alone to nurse with a bottle propped up on a pillow.

A baby can be nursed for two or three years if mother is healthy. Civilized women are too sophisticated to nurse that long, but the African mothers in underdeveloped areas often nurse for three years simply because the mortality rate is so high and the baby has a better chance with the natural immunization that is provided by the mother's milk.

It is my opinion that a baby should be nursed at least one year, and more if possible. It has never been my opinion to take a baby off of the breast and onto a cup. The nursing process should continue for at least 2 years. If taken off the breast, a bottle should be used. The ideas that a baby should go to a cup is an ego trip for a parent; it has nothing to do with benefit for the child. It is no wonder we have so many people sucking on pipes, cigars, cigarettes, and fingers, because they did not have enough sucking as a baby.

The bottle should be introduced right after birth with honey water and later fruit juice and herb teas, in order to make the transition easy when breast nursing is over. If the child does not take a bottle for the first two years, it is almost impossible to doctor them with herb teas, laxatives, vitamins, etc.

An idea prevalent lately, since doctors have again encouraged mothers to nurse, is that the child should have nothing but mother's milk. This conclusion has probably been drawn from studies regarding the feeding of baby cereals. The use of cereals has caused much pneumonia, colds, mucus, earaches, constipation, and bronchitis. Studies have shown that a baby cannot even digest any grains at that age.

The use of canned baby foods, including meat, with a great deal of sugar and salt, start a baby out with unnatural appetites as well as eating dead food with little or no food value.

If a baby is eating all cooked food, including bottle milk, it has little chance to be healthy. Science has proven that it requires the live enzymes in raw foods to transport the vitamins and minerals to the body cells. That is why it is so important to nurse.

Even though the baby may be nursing and receiving live enzymes, if the mother is not receiving adequate amounts of vitamins and minerals in her food, she is still not able to give such nutrients to her baby.

During pregnancy, as well as lactation, the baby will take all it can from the mother. When the mother does not have enough for baby and herself, it is always the mother who suffers the most. Some women lose their hair, teeth, fingernails, etc. during pregnancy and lactation. With this in mind, it pays to get the proper nutrition with lots of good, raw food.

How fresh is fresh food? This too, is an important factor. Is it organically grown? Is it heavily sprayed with poisons? All of these things must be considered for maximum health.

If a mother has good health, and is willing to eat correctly during pregnancy and while nursing, she should have an abundance of good milk to provide for her child. Fruit makes the richest and best milk. Watermelon is the fruit that makes the most milk.

If a lot of fruit is not available, alfalfa chlorophyll or alfalfa mint tea makes excellent milk, because of its high vitamin and mineral content. Carrot juice also makes good milk, because it, like alfalfa, has high calcium and all other minerals necessary to make calcium useable in the body.

The protein requirements for man are definitely proven by the changes occurring in the milk of the mother at different stages in the development of the child. It is interesting that the amount of protein diminishes as the baby grows older. Starting at birth with 2.38% protein and diminishing to 1.07% protein by six months of age.

The likely consequences for most babies fed on pasteurized cow's milk is that they not only do not get enough minerals, vitamins, and enzymes from dead milk, but they get too much protein. Cow's milk, by comparison to mother's milk, is 16% protein, which is far too much for human consumption. This could explain the many crib deaths due to suffocation caused from too high a protein, mucus forming milk. Cow's milk, if used, should be raw and diluted with water.

A better milk for humans, however, is raw goats milk. Some doctors in California are prescribing carrot juice for babies who develop too much mucus, bronchitis, or recurring pneumonia. A glass of carrot juice has much more calcium than a glass of milk and has all the component mineral and vitamins without the high protein. Carrot juice, however, lacks the fatty acids or oils so necessary to growth and development. A baby only needs about two to three bottles a day of carrot juice, but about 2 teaspoons of soft or unhydogenated oil must be added to the bottle. Apple juice or other fresh juices should be used at other feedings.

Apple juice can be given for all other feedings when using carrot juice, but citrus should be used only one feeding per day.

If digestion is poor, liquid acidophilus culture can be added to the bottle.

Babies have an enzyme called gastric lipase, which digests fat in the stomach. This lasts about three years, and is a good gauge as to how long a child should drink milk. A small amount of honey should be added to milk or water, but not fruit juice or carrot juice. Sugar should never be added to the baby's milk or food.

SOME TIPS FOR BABY ASTHMA AND COLIC

Baby asthma
Cayenne and water (weak solution) in eye dropper
(Then added to a small baby bottle of water)
Approx. 1,000 mg. Vitamin C (powdered can be taken with
    honey and water)
Approx. 2 ounce laxative tea
Enema - where fever is present
Relaxing herbs to calm baby:
    Hops tea and honey or
    Catnip tea and honey
To induce sleep:
    Chamomile tea and honey
No milk - only fruit juice or alfalfa mint tea during attack.
For Colic:
    Bayberry tea and honey or
    Alfalfa mint tea and honey or
    Ginger tea and honey or
No milk until attack subsides

Hot water bottle on stomach
To relax and help baby to sleep:
    Hops tea and honey
    Catnip tea and honey
    Chamomile tea and honey

In conclusion, the herbs, alfalfa and red raspberry, increase the flow of milk, while sage and parsley diminish the flow of milk, so they should only be used when weaning baby.

CHAPTER 4

CARE OF BABY FROM BIRTH TO TWO YEARS OLD

Mother has the most control over her baby's diet between birth and two years old. If her baby is ever sick, it is her fault. Even grandparents will usually not interfere with the feeding of the baby, unless he is left in their care. A baby is such a tender little treasure, that most grandparents are happy to let Mom and Dad make the decisions and take responsibility. Raising a baby from birth to two exacts a constant vigil on the part of his parents.

When children get a little older and more secure with life and living, if Mom and Dad have not been attentive, the child may not be liked very well by anyone as he reaches the terrible twos and begins to want things his way.

The first two years are the most precious and important to his future behavior and thought patterns. A child left to his own devices, or left with an unconcerned babysitter, will just learn by osmosis, soaking up everything that comes his way, good or bad. He will have no standard of excellence to reach for, with no one to teach him comparative values. Parents are foolish indeed, when they let these years slip by with no positive instruction and discipline.

A bond of love and obedience can be established at this period more than at any other time in the child's life. If a mother could give each child her undivided attention for three years, they would be the best years she could spend with him.

With so many mothers working full time, just to support the family, children and mothers both miss a special time in their lives. Even if mother has to work, or is a single parent, the time she spends with the child should be meaningful. She should still be concerned with what her baby eats when not in her care. A young woman I knew, who was a single parent, fixed all the good food her child was to eat each day, and took it to the sitter, with instructions that he was not to have anything else to eat but what she packed for him. A mother could provide books to be read to the child and all kinds of positive learning tools and toys, with instructions to the sitter as to nap time and planned play.

From birth to two years, a child is like a little piece of clay, soft, pliable, and easy to mold, but it takes time, patience, and love. Some people don't like children because they see them as a threat to their own wants and time. Good parents just get a kick out of the process of child raising and enjoy it.

A child learns faster, it seems, in this period, than at any other, going from not being able to talk, walk, or think much, to a toddling little person with his own personality.

There are parents who do not even like their own child until he turns into someone with whom they can communicate.

For vital health, a baby should be nursed for at least a year, and should be fed nothing else but raw fruit (blended in the blender), herb teas and honey, and fruit juices. After the first year, vegetables can be added to the diet, but the diet should still consist of more raw fruit than vegetables.

A child will develop his taste for wrong food at an early age, if they are introduced to him. By the same token, he will develop a taste for the right foods if that is what he is fed. The idea of putting sugar or salt in baby food is only to suit distorted adult tastes.

There are many parents, sad to say, who just tolerate children and whatever they do. Usually, this type of child is not welcome at anyone's house. My Dad, J.M. Gibby, wrote a little verse that applies here.

"Many people who credit themselves with tolerance, are in reality, only indifferent, for tolerance is based on love, understanding, and forgiveness, with a will to serve or assist. While indifference is based upon disregard, mental laziness, lack of will to oppose, or the spineless habit of following the line of least resistance."

Leah Widstoe, in her book, How to be Well, said:

"It is noble to help those who are ill and suffering, while trying to restore their health, but it is far nobler to teach one or a thousand how to build health so that suffering and disease may be prevented."

When we learn a better way to eat and live, the struggle begins, so it is far easier to start a child out on the right way early in life.

J.M. Gibby said:

'Every hardship we encounter in life, if conquered, is a great stepping stone toward our ultimate goal, whatever it may be. But unconquered, it remains a persistent stumbling block which impedes our progress until we develop the will and the intelligence to remove it from our path."

CHAPTER 5

HOW TO FEED THE GROWING CHILD, BUILD THE IMMUNE SYSTEM, AND AVOID CHILDHOOD DISEASES AND IMMUNIZATIONS

If you have read the chapter about how the body feeds and heals itself, you probably already know what I will tell you now.

When a mother and father wish to give their children the very best start in life, it is important for them to know the truth. Where do they go to find the truth in this world of so many half-truths and downright lies, many of which are told by unscrupulous men and women to get gain, no matter who it hurts?

After having raised six children by natural methods, only having to see a doctor to have a bone set or have a wound sewn, I can say, with all confidence, that it is much easier in the long run, as well as financially advantageous, to prevent illness, rather than try to restore health after it is gone.

If a mild food diet will heal terminal disease, why wouldn't it be the best way to prevent disease? When disease is understood, it is nothing more than the accumulation of uneliminated waste. If the average diet causes such accumulation of waste and has not the ability to remove it out of the body, and the mild food will cleanse it out, then the facts speak for themselves.

Not everyone wants perfect health. They would rather eat their cake and bare the pain, drink the alcohol, or smoke the cigarette. Some people would rather eat what they like, even if it kills them.

What do you want for your children? Do you want a better life physically for them, but are unwilling to set the example? Somehow, it does not work that way.

Throughout history, Mama has said, "Do as I say, not as I do." It is the same old story; abused children become abusing parents. Parents who pop drugs, smoke, and drink alcohol teach their children to become users, and often sooner than the parents had wished. Children whose parents do forbidden things can hardly wait until they are old enough to try it also.

Apart from all of this, the situation boil down to, what do you want for yourself and your family? Is the price of pain worth the pleasure derived from what ever you want, which breaks the laws of nature? You must decide.

You can go a little way and no improvement. You can go half way and be surprised, or you can try for the best. It is up to you. Learning this truth could save you thousands of dollars in doctor bills, not to mention pain and suffering. If you do not have a serious disease, you could jump back and forth from correct diet to incorrect, until you proved it to yourself.

Having established my position, I challenge you to prove the method right or wrong. I have proven it to myself over and over for some fifty years and found it always to be true.

Knowing a truth and living it - that is the problem. Knowing the laws of nature can be one of the greatest blessings of life, if you can live by the rules. I did not make the rules; I have only found them through much suffering and prayer.

If you want your children to be healthy and beautiful, you will feed them as much mild food as possible and as much raw food as possible. Even at best, someone is liable to come along and feed your child junk food. If you can keep your child's body free from toxic waste, clean and beautiful inside and out, the immune system of the body will work continually in its defense. The child will be happy and will learn at a remarkable rate.

So many children today, have overloaded their systems beyond their ability to function. Some go around biliously in a daze, half asleep, not able to live life to its fullest. Many children are filled with so much sugar, they become so hyper, that no one can stand them. Their nervous systems are wracked with pain. So what do the teachers do? Send a note home which says, "Have Johnny see his doctor and give him something. I can't cope with him in class." Then what does the doctor do? He gives him uppers or downers, as the problem demands, just like he will find on the street in a few years.

For the times mother needs to help her child over acute illness, the following are some helpful suggestions and alternatives to the use of drugs.

Note how many things vitamin C is useful for and how many diseases and symptoms are caused from the lack of it. All young mothers should become acquainted with vitamin C. A growing child should have no less than 1,000 mg. a day, and when sick, no less than 8,000 mg. a day, taken 1,000 mg. an hour.

Vitamin C necessary for:
cell respiration
breaking down protein
healing
capillary
cartilage and connective tissue

Vitamin C useful in:
aspirin poisoning
snake bites

black widow spider bites
poison oak or ivy
carbon monoxide poisoning
radiation poisoning
broken bones
bruises
burns
poisonous bites

Useful in acute disease:
meningitis
encephalitis
virus disease
swollen glands
 polio
 asthma
respiratory
acute sinus
kidney infection
croup
nose bleeding
promotes blood clotting
metal poisoning
hay fever
colds
virus diseases (mumps, measles, chicken pox)
sore throat, strep
phlebitis
inflamation

Symptoms of the lack of Vitamin C
anemia
bleeding membrane (mouth, red toothbrush)
low blood pressure
nosebleed
loose teeth
edema
wounds will not heal

pigmentation during pregnancy
varicose veins
hepatitis, liver
cataracts
glaucoma
high blood pressure
ulcers
arthritis, gout
weakness in arteries
cold sores
adrenal exhaustion
rheumatic fever
high cholesterol
mononucleosis
disc problems

There has been much discussion about vitamin C. It has been my experience and the experience of many others, that when vitamin C is used (1,000 mg. an hour) in acute illness, such as a cold, etc., it dissolves mucus and usually stops acute disease or inflamation within a day or two. It has been used successfully even with small babies.

Vitamin C has been considered to be harmful to the kidney when taken in high doses. Certainly it is when it is a coal tar product. Taking high doses of coal tar would be harmful. To determine whether or not your vitamin C is a coal tar product, you can make this experiment. Place the tablet or powder on a teaspoon with water, hold it over the burner of the stove, and let it boil. If it boils away to a white powder, it is not a coal tar product. If it boils to a sticky, black gum, it is a coal tar product. Vitamin C has recently been made from wood, and of course, would be a synthetic. When made from corn and citrus, it is a natural food product. When used in case of a cold or acute disease, it should be determined just how the vitamin C you use is made, or you will not get the results. Could this be the reason for the controversy about vitamin C? I have found, where acute disease is present, straight ascorbic acid is best, usually taking it only a day or two, as it dissolves mucus rapidly. Any acute disease brings with it rapid pulse, as waste is on the move in the blood. High doses of vitamin C often increase the heartbeat, as with acute disease. The addition of approximately one single O capsule of cayenne, will usually slow down and smooth out the heart. Bioflavonoid vitamin C is best for daily dose.

With twenty-five 500 mg. tablets, liquified, with 1/8 cup warm water, each teaspoon will equal 1,000 mg; add honey to taste. Polio virus has been stopped in 72 hours with vitamin C therapy. We have too long starved the diabetic of fruit sugars and accompanying vitamin C, which could stop the inflamation and running ulcers that seem to go with later stages of diabetes.

Vitamin C is actually an aid to saving the kidneys, as it keeps the mucus or inflamation from causing damage, dissolves the mucus, thus allowing it to pass through the kidneys. Bright's disease or any kidney damage is usually caused from a bad inflamation or acute disease, with too much mucus passing through the kidneys, causing a break or damage to the filtering system of the kidney. When used in conjunction with herbs for the kidneys, and where there has been previous damage, vitamin C is not damaging to the kidneys as has been thought. It may also be interesting to note that you can start an elimination by taking high doses of vitamin C, bringing on a cold. When vitamin C is taken in large doses, for extended periods, such as five to ten days, calcium and vitamin B should be added, as the vitamin C leaches these elements and causes nervousness.

Young mothers should also become knowledgeable about the use of enemas. An enema can bring down a fever within about fifteen minutes.

FEVER

Fever is nature's way of bringing impurities to the surface and is also nature's way of warning that all systems are clogged, and help is needed immediately. A fever has been described as a car running with its brakes on. Fever only occurs when other channels of elimination are not removing waste material fast enough, or when they are stopped. Again, do as with the common cold: help nature.

Usually, an enema will bring the fever right down. Vitamin C, fruit, and many herbs will assist in such cases. Goldenseal root is antibiotic and helps to kill germs. It is good to keep the body covered and warm. Cayenne is exceptionally good when irregularity of the heart exists or when it beats too fast. The heart will always beat faster during a disease crisis, or when taking high doses of vitamin C.

In case of fever, take an enema, treat as for a cold, and give sponge baths with cool water when the temperature gets too high (104 degrees). All acute disease can be treated in a similar way as a cold.

ENEMA

The enemas given in the hospitals are a disgrace, causing the constipation you have noticed, after an operation or having a baby. They pump two quarts of water into the lower descending colon and tell you to hold it no matter what impaction may be in the descending colon, thus distending the lower bowel. What happens to a balloon when you blow it up? Yes, it loses its elasticity, and that is exactly what happen when the lower colon is distended by two quarts of water. Then as the waste matter from above moves down, it fills up the larger distended area, closing smaller at the anus, rather than being moved out; matter will then usually stay and harden and have constipation.

The correct way to take an enema is to first of all lie on the left side. Make sure the hose is free of air bubbles by allowing it to run some water through first. Insert tip, allowing warm water to run in until the least cramp is felt, then expel. Keep doing this continually, introducing water and expelling it even if you have to do it over and over many times, a little at a time, until water reaches the waistline. Then turn on the back, continuing in the same way, cleaning the transverse colon. When water has reached the waist at the right side, turn over on to the right side and clean the ascending side. By the time the entire colon has been cleaned in this way, usually taking in the process, two full bags, a little at a time, the third bag will usually go the entire length of the colon and the water expelled will be clear.

Warm water at first, relaxes and causes less cramping. Cool water tones, like astringent and is best in the last water taken.

There is in use in some hospitals a drug solution in a small amount which effects an evacuation. This amount of fluid to give an enema does not distend the lower bowel as much, but what does the drug do to the bowel?

By the time your child is eight years old, he should know how and be able to give himself an enema. He should have been accustomed to enemas since he was a baby and never frightened by it. I have known of grown men who were terrified at the prospect of taking an enema.

Listed below are most of the major acute diseases common to the average family and what can be done for them without drugs.

COMMON COLD

The common cold is nature's way to save a life. If you eat wrong and say, AI never have a cold", there is usually a chronic toxic condition in the head area. A cold is nature's way of cleaning your house so you can continue life. When your body builds toxic waste to a dangerous point - if you have good vitality - your body will force a disease crisis, anything from a cold to the flu, all virus diseases, or contagious diseases. You will always feel better after the crisis than before. Nature, at this time does not always clean down to immaculate cleanliness. Nature only cleans until nutrition is again required to maintain your body strength, then soon may force another crisis and clean some more. This is why you may keep having one cold after another, or have pneumonia two or three times. Of course the thing we usually do as soon as our house has been swept a little is to fill it again with unnatural toxic foods. It is like sweeping trash out one door as fast as you sweep it in the other. You can never get ahead of it.

COLD

Enema, laxative, or both
Approximately 1,000 mg. vitamin C each hour
No food except fruit and fruit juices
Tonic teas:
    Comfrey
    Red Clover
    Alfalfa mint
    Horse Tail

ECZEMA

Vitamin C: at least 4,000 mg. per day
Chia: soak in warm water until thick, place on affected area to
    stop pain. As pain returns, change poultice.
Clean blood by changing diet to mild food
Clean bowels with enema and laxative
Check laundry soap

EARACHE

Ice bag on ear scatters the inflammation, relieving pain in about
    fifteen minutes or less.
Feet in hot mustard or cayenne water
Enema
Stop eating, except fruit and juice
Approx. 1,000 mg. vitamin C per hour
Laxative teas draw mucus from the ear:
    Horsetail
    Juniper (for kidneys)
    Alfalfa

MEASLES

Measles can be avoided, like all other contagious disease, if the
body is clean and well-nourished (see section on common cold, use
same methods). There are many herbs which will help in case of
measles, either to bring the breaking-out into full bloom, or to help
after breaking-out has occurred. Saffron tea, taken quite warm, (never

boil) will cause a break-out if measles are suspected and fever persists after an enema. Also the juice of a boiled grapefruit rind or alfalfa mint tea helps. A soda bath helps to alkalize the skin. To soothe the itching child, a warm catnip enema is helpful. You can give him a tea using approx. 1 tsp. pleurisy root and approx.1 tsp. ginger; steep this in boiled water. (Never boil herbs - steep only) Camomile tea, vervain, yarrow, and lady slipper, may also be used.

BOILS (Rash, Pimples, etc.)

These are caused from too much mucus in the blood, eliminating through the skin when the bowel and kidneys are not performing well. The skin is often affected when there is adrenal insufficiency. Asthmatics often tend to skin rash, due to inability to cope with stress. However, without the mucus in the lung, there would not be an asthma attack.

VIRUS DISEASE
(Measles, Mumps, Chicken Pox, Smallpox, Pneumonia, Polio, Typhoid)

Stop eating concentrated foods
Eat fruit and fruit juice only
Take herb laxative and enema
Vitamin C - approx. 1,000 - 2,000 mg. per hour
Hot saffron tea or boiled grapefruit rind and fruit (strain and drink hot) to help break-out when fever is high
Wild carrot
Use same method as with a cold

INFLAMMATION

Cayenne: 1 "oo" capsule each hour until pain is gone
Alfalfa mint tea, up to one cup each hour
Bowel: take laxative herbs
Throat: mix glycerin and iodine until glycerin becomes a deep amber color. Swab throat every hour. Even a serious strep throat will respond to this method.

Eyes: make eyewash of goldenseal root and bayberry, strain through paper towel. Use eyecup or dropper.

BURNS

Another problem while raising a family occurs at some time in all households, is what to do for a burn.

Initial treatment:
Cold water or ice until pain stops and area is cooled

Any of the following:
Vitamin E oil
Comfrey (raw, bruised, and added to a small amount of water in blender and made into a poultice)
Aloe vera (bruised and put directly on burn)
Powdered comfrey
Powdered goldenseal root
Follow up:
Vitamin B complex (approx. 4 tablets) and calcium (approx. 4 tablets) to help the child sleep after the shock of a burn. To avoid infection of a serious burn, mix vitamin E oil and goldenseal root together in a soft paste and apply to burn. Goldenseal root is the antibiotic, and vitamin E is the healer.

WOUNDS

Cuts, scrapes, and puncture wounds can also be treated in a natural way without drugs.

Cuts and scrapes will both respond well to powdered goldenseal root sprinkled directly on the wound and then bandaged. Even if the wound is serious enough to have stitches, goldenseal root can be used with each changing of the bandage. You will be amazed at how fast it heals.

Puncture wounds should be treated a little differently than other wounds. Make it bleed freely if possible, and use method as with a cold for two or three days. Use goldenseal root internally and directly on the wound.

BRUISES AND BUMPS

Bruises and bumps respond best to fresh tobacco as a poultice (the only good use for tobacco), or comfrey poultice. Comfrey is excellent taken internally for inward bruises, and also has bone-knitting qualities.

BEE STINGS

Bee stings and burns both respond to nettle externally, but nettle can be taken in a tea form for bee sting and helps to flush out the poison. Vitamin C in high doses, depending on the poison, can save a lot of sickness, even with snake bite. It must be taken in extreme dosage, (2,000 - 3,000 mg.) Every half hour for a few hours, then 1,000 mg. and hour, until poison is eliminated. Then use method as with a cold, using no heavy foods. Take a laxative and an enema and eat only fruit until poison is gone.

NOSEBLEED

A nosebleed can be stopped immediately by taking a 2 to 1/3 tsp of cayenne in water for a child 5 years or older, up to 1 tsp. for adults. Cayenne powder put directly on a heavily bleeding wound will stop the bleeding immediately.

NATURAL IMMUNIZATION

It is believed, in most natural circles, that immuntization is unnecessary, if the body is kept in a clean and well nourished state. Mothers who believe this, have difficulty with school officials. The greatest concern with schools who are federally funded, is that children will be absent, and they will lose money. Children who are properly nourished, are not among those who get a communicable disease or other sickness that would cause absenteeism. The school officials do not understand this.

It should be the prerogative of any person to decide if they are to be medicated, not the state or the federal government. The state health department often leads the way however, in a media coercion to force parents to have their children immunized. It was announced in the newspaper that a massive program to increase immunization of children one to fifteen years of age against preventable disease was under way as part of a campaign stated by the Department of Health, Education, and Welfare. Dr. Lyman J. Olsen, Utah division of Health director, stated that 100% immunization cannot be reached, since some parents will not allow children to receive shots for religious or for medical reasons, but that the purpose of the program was to prevent outbreaks of the diseases.

Another part of the program was to establish a permanent system to ensure that all children born in Utah every year are immunized. A survey of all children, to identify susceptible children who have not been immunized was to be made, then a "knock on doors", to encourage parents to arrange for shots. Also, distribution of information was to be made through the news media, government agencies and other organizations.

In Mena, Arkansas, the son and two daughters of a farmer were vaccinated by order of the Arkansas Supreme Court, climaxing long court battles on the issue of state vs. religion. The children had not attended school for six years, since vaccinations are required by the school boards before they can enter. The father believed that vaccinations are against the will of God, but the judge ruled that he could not deny the children an education on religious grounds, and they were forcibly vaccinated. It would seem they had it backwards: it was the government denying the education, not the father.

In San Antonio, Texas, it was reported that a Private, James B. Merritt, had written asking his senator for help in avoiding a polio shot after having gone to the offices of the Secretary of the Army and been refused. He stated he would rather be shot with a .45 than to have the immunization shots, since it is against his religious beliefs, but the army ordered him to take the polio shot anyway.

Dr. Harry Gibbons of the Salt Lake City, County Health Department, stated that students could be expelled from school starting in December 1978, if they didn't have their immunization shots. He regrets, that despite efforts of various health official and school administrators, some parents have refused to have their children immunized, but his department has responsibility for enforcing the state law that requires school children to be immunized for mumps, rubella, diphtheria, tetanus, pertussis, and polio, as well as measles.

This sort of coercion is freely put out in the media, even when the law clearly states that a person has the right to refuse inoculation.

The paper reported that the Davidson County, Tennessee Grand Jury indicted a father of two on a misdemeanor because he refused to allow his children to be immunized with polio shots. Was this true or just more propaganda scare tactics to make every child have his shots?

Elizabeth W. Shafer, in a letter to the editor in 1979, stated that the paper should stop making false statements about required immunizations to enter school. She said that there are provisions in the law for those opposed to immunization, and people should not be intimidated. There is plenty of evidence as to the harm of these shots, but the controlled media will not print them. She states that they will try to stop a compulsory bill past the freedom loving people one of these days.

Two years later, she wrote to the editor of the Ogden newspaper again, stating that we go through it every fall. The paper publishes that immunization is required by law for school entry and day care centers. The State Public Health service said they had not made such a statement and blamed the media. She believes the medical profession and drug interests would like it to be compulsory.

There are articles from time to time, pro and con, such as a story from England, reported in the Ogden Standard Examiner, Jan. 6, 1977. A London labor party lawmaker, Jack Ashley, was trying to get compensation from the government for victims of immunizations that went wrong. He said that happy, healthy babies had been turned into cabbages within a few days of their DPT immunizations. Three hundred children had suffered brain damage, blindness, deafness, or paralysis.

Some medical authorities stated they thought the children could have been among those predisposed to brain disorders and were just triggered by the vaccination and stated that whooping cough sometimes causes brain damage.

The British Medical Association said they believed that the benefits of the vaccine far outweighed any side effects, claiming that before mass immuntization was introduced in Britain in the 1950's, there was an average of 160 child deaths each year from whooping cough, and that had now dropped to only two a year.

In May 1976, the paper reported that according to the director of the communicable disease section of the Utah State Health Division, too many children who have been vaccinated against the measles are getting them. Efforts have been made to determine if the virus is different from that in the vaccine. He hoped the epidemic of the disease would let up now, since it had started almost a year ago, and he was encouraging parents to immunize their children even though it did not assure protection.

Health officials in Des Moines Iowa, were puzzled over the sudden polio epidemic that hit their city. It recorded 71 polio cases, the last two of them with the dreaded bulbar type, had not received the Salk vaccine. However, there had been a survey to show that while the Blacks were the hardest hit, they had received an equal proportion of the Salk shots to the whites.

In September 1978, Atlanta reported that health officials in eleven states were asked by the National Center for Disease Control to stop administering a vaccine while reactions by 24 children were being investigated.

The DPT vaccine is used to immunize against diphtheria, whooping cough, and tetanus. This evidently caused some children to develop marble-sized lumps on their arms, unusual swelling and redness, pain, fever, and discomfort that lasted several days. It was stressed that the reaction was not "life threatening", and none of those affected were hospitalized.

In August 1980, the Salt Lake City-County Health officials said, that children will not be allowed to register for kindergarten this year unless they had been immunized. The school districts and private schools in the area would help enforce this requirement. Children transferring from out of state, will be allowed a thirty day grace period to secure records or their immunization.

Because of propaganda on the news media, radio, TV, and newspapers, when I sent a note to school refusing to have my son inoculated, and left for a lecture in California, I fully expected to come home and find him expelled from school. He was not, however, and looking into the law, I could see they could not expel him.

Rights of a free people cannot be sacrificed by mass medication, simply to keep the school support rolling in, or for any other reason.

A man speaking on the floor at a Utah hearing, said he did not want the people who would not have their children inoculated to be carriers to his children. This is a ridiculous argument that school nurses always gave me about my children. My answer would be, "Do you believe the vaccines really work?" Their answer was always a definite, "yes". So I would return with, "If all the other children have their shots, they do not have to worry about getting anything from my children".

Most of my children were raised without the shots and did not contract the childhood diseases. My oldest son almost died from an inoculation, so I felt I had the right of refusal on all of my other children.

It has always been my belief, that if the body is kept clean, there is no need to fear the microbe. Therefore, after being coerced into having my oldest son inoculated, which nearly caused his death, my other children were not ever inoculated for anything. Living on a clean, mucusless diet, none of them ever got the childhood diseases. One of my daughters got the mumps at age 18, during the dating years of junk food diet. She asked me why she didn't get the mumps when she was a child. I told her, "when you were a child, I was taking care of you, now you are an adult, you are taking care of yourself, and not doing a very good job".

Vaccination has always been a political problem, not a medical one. The states depending on the federal money only receive money when the children are in school, so their fear is that contagion will cause too much absenteeism. There are a number of books on the market discouraging parents from inoculation and showing the dangers. A number of current newspaper articles have disclosed apparent danger much more than the diseases the shots are designed to prevent. Even if a child dies because of the shots, or develops the disease after inoculation, the parents have no recourse except to sue the powerful chemical company who made the drug.

Preventative, natural methods, are the answer, if parents are willing to take the time and the effort to see that their children eat wholesome, clean food.

CHAPTER 6

ACUTE CHILDHOOD DISEASES

COMMON COLD

Definition and pathology of Natural healing does not differ with medical science as to definition, with the exception that a cold or any acute disease is only contagious when the body is toxic enough for the germs to live and multiply. When the body is clean, the microbe cannot and does not start an elimination of waste. Some scientists believe now that we have all of the microbes waiting dormant in our bodies or remain useful in some other functions until the immune system breaks down. This is close to my belief. Soon science will have to discover with that beginning, that the immune system is maintained by correct eating habits and clean nourishing food, and that nature kills the weak, undernourished body by the use of parasites and germs to bring the body back to dust. We have known and watched this process in plants, where the weak ones develop bugs and die. Man even tries to build a sound, healthy body using plants that are raised chemically, lacking in enough strength to avoid being killed by bugs. He then foolishly sprays the bugs with poison and eats the weak plant. He somehow expects his own immune system to be strong when the food he eats is already weak. This is why it is important to eat organically grown food that has been properly nourished.

When enough germs are present and enough waste has been accumulated to interfere with normal functions, the body forces the waste into the bloodstream, causing a rise in temperature, swollen glands, sore throat, and related symptoms. Pain then follows, when too much waste fills the blood and the white count is elevated or appears to be. It has been supposed, that the white cell combats infection and is a necessity. I say, there has to be something wrong with the white count theory, since in acute or chronic conditions, as the body begins its process of detoxification, the white count goes up, and after the cleanse, the white count goes down and the red count goes up. Science has taken that to believe that the white is necessary to fight infection. I believe it is there only to act as a holding cell until waste can be moved while the process is going on, and if a body were extremely clean, there would be little accumulation of white cells. We know that as the chronic person begins to cleanse naturally, the white count goes extremely high, and as the body becomes completely detoxified, the white count goes down and the red count goes up.

When I was at the Livingston Cancer Clinic, with Virginia Livingston, I saw graphs, which showed a lowered number of white cells, when using fruit juice in the diet. The assumption was that fruit juice was not as good for cancer nutrition because it cut down on the white cells that combat against the disease.

When I know that cancer and all other acute or terminal disease can be overcome with a fruitarian diet, there must be something wrong with the white cell theory as we know it.

Virus disease and pneumonia, are more violent than a cold in their cleansing process, so their related microscopic organisms are more powerful in their action. If a person were to develop the plague in a very toxic body, its cleansing action would kill within three days. Like pneumonia, it cleans quickly down to clean or dead.

Measles, mumps, chicken pox, and all acute disease can be avoided upon exposure, if the body is clean. To believe that older people have fewer colds because they have had more time to build immunity, is a mistaken idea medical science fosters. A child's ability to throw off waste is strong and the young and old develop chronic disease unto death, because their ability to throw off waste has been diminished. When children die young, it is because their bodies lack the youthful ability to throw off the waste, or they have accumulated more waste than they can throw off, becoming chronic unto death. Sometimes, as has happened in the last 20 years of drug use and abuse, children are born with organic deformities, so their ability to detoxify does not function properly.

NATURAL TECHNIQUE

An enema and a laxative are the first things to remember in treatment of a cold or acute disease. A cold is not caught, it is earned, by wrong eating habits - too much concentrated foods and too much protein. To overcome a cold, it is necessary to clean the body quickly. A cold is Nature's process to save life. When a cold begins, and the body is changed from a feeding organ, to an eliminative organ, eating only prolongs the misery.

It has been known for many years among health enthusiasts, that a cold can be overcome quickly, within a few days, if nature is helped in her process, by stopping the intake of all food, except fruit and fruit juice, herb teas, lemon and honey. The reason for this is that the body, at the time of a cold, is forcing as much toxic waste as possible into the bloodstream for evacuation. Cold germs are merely the vehicle which starts the process of elimination in order to rid the body of waste which could otherwise interfere with the function of vital organs. Germs do not live on sound, healthy tissue, but on the waste of the body. A cold is a blessing. All the germs in the world could not cause a cold if the body were clean. I tell my classes to "enjoy a cold, you earned it". Behold the wonder that nature performs in your behalf, when you do not obey her rules! A good cold will buy you more time, so you can continue to live.

Germs trigger acute disease, but parasites and microbes live in chronic disease, adding their waste to the refuse of the body in which they live.

HELPFUL AIDS DURING A COLD

Fruits are the highest in glucose sugar and ascorbic acid, in marvelous combination. They, therefore, serve as the best food for an acute cleanse. Using fruits, along with the addition of vitamin C (Approx. 1,000 - 2,000 mg. an hour, each waking hour), expedites the process and accelerates it to a few days rather than one to three weeks required to overcome a cold while continuing to eat. Vitamin C seems to dissolve the mucus and waste and carry it out through the kidneys. Vitamin C does not stop the process of elimination, causing waste to eventually turn into chronic disease, as often occurs with aspirin and other repressive drugs.

Niacin or Vitamin B-3, is useful when taken with vitamin C to remove mucus waste from the head area. Approximately 100 mg. daily, 50 mg. at a time.

HERBS HELPFUL FOR A COLD

Senna, Cascara Sagrada: or any good laxative herbal formula is good. It is important to use laxative herbs first. A laxative and enema will lower fever quickly, because when the bowel is full, the waste on the move in the bloodstream cannot be eliminated. The body therefore does the next best thing, and forces it out through the skin in the form of fever.

Echinacea, poke root, burdock, and coltsfoot: are good for swollen glands and for a general cleansing of the body.

Elderberries, rosehips, and watercress: have all been used with great success for colds and fever, either in a tea or powder form. Watercress is the first cleansing herb to grow in the spring.

Alfalfa mint tea: is always useful, especially when the person cannot take a lot of vitamin C. In cases where uric acid levels or lactic acid levels are extreme, as in hypoglycemia, vitamin C caused irritation in the stomach. Such people do well on alfalfa and liquid chlorophyll, to alkalize their body in place of vitamin C. They can also use rosehips as a high source of natural vitamin C.

Goldenseal root: also has alkaline attributes, but is used more as an antibiotic for colds and viruses. Approximately 5 - 6 Aoo" size capsules a day, taken 2 hours apart, can be beneficial.

Cayenne: is also used for fever and is most helpful. Cayenne is high in natural vitamin C.

Calcium lactate and/or chlorophyll: can be used with vitamin C as a buffer where the vitamin C is irritating. The vitamin C is then tolerated.

Assist nature: rest, lots of liquids, herb teas, and fruit juice or lemon and honey.

Garlic or goldenseal root: can be used in the enema to kill germs and worms. Use approximately 1 tsp. goldenseal root or 1 chopped clove of fresh garlic. Soak garlic in hot water until water is cool, strain and pour into enema bag, add warm water to correct water temperature.

For Chest congestion and swollen glands or headache, combine equal parts of:
    Eucalyptus oil
    Peppermint oil
    Camphorated oil
    Wintergreen oil
Apply to chest or glands as needed

All acute disease, inflamation, or infection will respond to these techniques for overcoming a cold

    .

PREVENTATIVE MEASURES

Maintain high vitamin and mineral intake on a permanent basis, as well as daily doses of vitamin C. Keep the system clean and free of accumulated waste, by eating more fruits and vegetables, fewer concentrated foods such as starch, meats, dairy products, and sugars. Eat food higher in natural glucose sugar and vitamin C, such as fruit.

CROUP

Treat as for a cold, but for immediate relief, use straight lemon and honey, approximately one spoonful at a time, every 15 minutes, until throat clears. Use a cold, wet wash cloth around the neck with a dry towel over it. Change and cool wash cloth often to keep neck cold until swelling goes down.

DIPHTHERIA

The membrane that fuels the throat can be quickly dissolved with straight lemon and honey. As soon as possible, a strong laxative, followed two hours later by an enema with warm water and 2 tsp. goldenseal root in the water. Alfalfa mint tea and fruit juice, with no solid food for 3 - 4 days. When sore throat and fever leaves, solid food , in the form of fruit only, for another 3 days, then mild food until completely recovered.

Goldenseal root: approx. 1 - 3 capsules daily for 3 days
Vitamin C: 1,000 - 2,000 mg. an hour for 3 - 4 days
Lemon juice and honey (straight): approx. 1 spoonful
    every half hour

Cayenne, Lobelia, and Myrrh: in water (strong solution)
    gargle 2 - 3 times daily

HEADACHE

Headache is a symptomatic reflection of toxic waste constipation somewhere in the body. In most cases, it is caused by constipation of the bowel, large or small intestines, or both. A good laxative and an enema will usually stop the pain of a headache without taking drugs. Occasionally, a headache can be caused by the atlas or axis vertebra being out of place in the neck. A good chiropractic adjustment will often stop the pain.

EARACHE

My definition of earache, differs somewhat from medical science in that it is not an infection caused by a virus. Rather, the virus is the result of toxic waste in the region of the neck, head, and ears. The virus merely activates an elimination, allowing the body to rid itself of the waste.

Sometimes, infection elimination develops to the point of a bulge in the ear drum, and pain is an intense throbbing. The drum can burst, and will for certain, if heat is applied as medical science suggests. The break of inflamation can go back into the brain and cause death. If it is going to break, it would be better to break outwardly and drain. Many ruptures of the drum can cause scar tissue or the drum may not heal well, leaving a hole where water and other elements can enter, causing more infection and irritation. Deafness can result from scar tissue, or, as in some cases, the drum gradually disintegrates, requiring plastic surgery.

Method: an ice bag on the ear, rather than heat, is the best and fastest way to relieve pain so that the inflamation can be scattered. You would not put heat on an appendicitis, why would you put it on an ear infection, drawing the waste to a head and breaking the drum?

Feet in hot mustard or cayenne water helps to draw inflammation
    from the head area
Enema
Stop eating. Eat only fruit and drink juices
Vitamin C: approx. 1,000 mg. per hour

Herbs:
A strong laxative tea flushes the lymphatic system, pulling
    inflammation away from the head area
Horsetail tea or
Juniper tea or
Alfalfa mint tea, act to help the body flush waste through the
    kidneys.

CHICKEN POX

Definition: small reddish spots that appear on any part of the body, usually beginning on the chest and abdomen. Spots begin as pinpoint in size, becoming larger and spreading further and finally forming into blisters. As blisters heal, itching becomes bothersome. If scabs are pulled off, scarring takes place. Unless there is a toxic condition, in which Herpes Zoster virus can be activated, it is not possible to get chickenpox. If a toxic condition is suspected and the child has been exposed, begin healing procedure immediately, and the chickenpox can be avoided entirely or just a minor case with a few pox and no fever.

It is a childhood eliminative disease that is not necessary, if a child's body is kept clean and free of toxins.

NATURAL TECHNIQUE

Beginning upon exposure or fever, stop intake of all concentrated food or mild food. Drink alfalfa mint tea and honey, or warm lemon and honey water, fruit juices only for three days, then add solid fruit for three days, then add mild foods.

Enema using catnip tea
Herbal laxative

If fever is high, and chickenpox are suspected, but do not break out, hot saffron tea will make them pop right out. The sooner the pox break out, the quicker the disease will be overcome. The disease will have little discomfort if high doses of vitamin C are added to the diet. The same as with a cold, approximately 1,000 - 2,000 mg. every waking hour for three days. When glands are swollen, goldenseal root can be used, approximately 2 - 5 capsules a day for three days. Burdock root, yellow dock, and goldenseal root are helpful for itching, made into a tea and bathed on the sores.

BABY ENEMA

Use small ear syringe or baby syringe. Fill glass with warm water, empty syringe of all air, insert in glass of water and release syringe to fill the water into the syringe. Insert syringe into baby and squeeze the bulb. While still compressed remove the syringe from the baby. Follow same procedure about three times and allow time for the baby to expel the water each time. This will usually bring on evacuation and will bring a fever down within a few minutes.

CHAPTER 7

CHRONIC CHILDHOOD DISEASES

ASTHMA

Definition and pathology: In natural healing, asthma is one of the easiest diseases to overcome, provided the person is willing to change his or her diet. Often, a personality type is involved. A worrier or perfectionist type, who creates stressful daily situations is unable to produce enough adrenal hormones to cope with the stress they themselves produce. It is interesting that the adrenal hormones are required to utilize starch and meat, much the same as insulin helps in the ability to use sugar, changing sucrose to glucose by the time it reaches the small intestines and is absorbed into the blood stream for use.

If a person is eating too much starch and meat, and maintains a stressful lifestyle, there will not be enough adrenal hormone to go around. The body's first reaction, is to go into adrenal exhaustion, forcing the body to rest. There are several types of adrenal exhaustion, and each responds in a certain way to similar problem.

The asthmatic response: Hard breathing
Arthritic response: Building uric acid, holding calcium in the joints
Low blood sugar: Weak, hypoglycemia
Insanity: Certain types

Addison's disease: builds uric acid, but loses calcium, builds lactic acid in the abdominal cavity, increased weight, or weight loss with no lactic acid build up (fatigue in both types)

Skin Pigmentation

When the response to stress is asthmatic, other symptoms are not necessarily involved until in later life all adrenal exhaustion symptoms may become apparent. Usually, however, the person who is asthmatic, has certain physical appearances not noted in the other types. They may have a short diaphragm and indentation below the sternum. This physical feature seems to be noted at birth or early childhood and shows up on babies who have asthma. Whether or not this type is born with certain personality traits, developing the stress factor in infancy, or whether they are born with an organic inability to produce enough adrenal stress hormone is a question still to be answered.

NATURAL TECHNIQUE

Stop the intake of all toxic, mucus forming foods and food which drains and overworks the adrenals. Use the mild food diet. Listed below are adult doses; children 9 - 14 use 1/2 dose, children 2 - 8 use 1/3 dose.

Lung formula: Approx. 2 capsules daily needed in an acute attack.
>Mullein: 1 part (for magnesium and potassium)
>Comfrey: 1 part (loosens mucus, stops hemorrhaging)
>Marshmallow: 1 part (soothes inflamation, diuretic)
>Lobelia: 2 part (relaxant)

Take an enema
Stop eating solid foods until breathing is normal
Lobelia extract:
>Lobelia - 2 ounces
>Cayenne - 2 ounces
>Apple cider or malt vinegar - 1 ounce

Allow to stand 10 days. Shake often, daily, strain after 10 days, and then bottle for use. Approximately 1 tsp. lobelia extract in water will usually cause vomiting. Extract is usually used at night, where the asthma attack is caused from food ingested at the night meal which has not emptied from the stomach. When the stomach is empty, normal breathing will usually return. If it does not, because of a cold, continue vitamin C and lung formula. The usual response with the lung formula is relief and normal breathing in 15 minutes. Even in extreme conditions, normal breathing will last several hours before the lung formula needs to be repeated.

Vitamin C is used only where there is a condition of a cold. It dissolves mucus, moves waste out quickly through the kidneys, and also neutralizes acids. Vitamin C should be used in an on going process after the acute condition is overcome. Use approximately 3,000 - 5,000 mg. daily as a preventative. Approximately 1,000 - 2,000 mgs. Every hour during acute condition.

Licorice root powder acts on the adrenals. Take approximately 2 - 4 capsules daily, continually allowing the person to better handle stress. Licorice acts like a cortisone in one respect, since it seems to overcome the feeling of stress. Unlike cortisone, it does not force the glands to produce hormones; rather, it acts as if the person had produced it themselves and uses it much the way insulin and other animal gland substances act in the body. It does not become addictive. As the body begins to heal, with corrective diet, the need for additional licorice root diminishes and if stopped instantly, would not cause any withdrawal symptoms. Within a relatively short time, all attacks of hard breathing will become a thing of the past, unless the person goes back to occasionally indulging in toxic, mucus forming foods.

Nervine Formula #1: 2 "o" size capsules daily for children under 12, twice as much for adults (relaxes the nervous system)
    Lady Slipper: 1 part
    Valerian: 1 part
    Mistletoe: 1/8 part
    Hops: 1/4 part

Black Cohosh: 1/8 part
Wood Betony: 1/8 part
Lobelia: 1/8 part
Scullcap: 1 part
Goldenseal Root: 2 part

Nervine Formula #2: approx. 2 - 3 "o" size capsules daily for children under 12, twice as much for adults. Useful in epileptic conditions or just to sleep well. (all the herbs listed below are nervine, relaxant, herbs, and in combination, make an excellent tranquilizer)

Equal parts of:
   Valerian
   Scullcap
   Lady Slipper
   Catnip
   Red Clover
Multi vitamin
Multi mineral
B complex: approx. 2 - 4 tablets daily acts as a relaxant, and heals the nervous system
Calcium: approx. 4 - 6 tablets daily

BABY ASTHMA

Cayenne and water (weak solution in eye dropper under tongue)
Vitamin C: Approx. 1,000 mg. an hour for acute attack
Herbal laxative tea: about 2 ounce
Give an enema where fever is present
Use herbs in a tea for relaxing and calming the baby:
   Hops or catnip tea and honey to induce sleep
   Chamomile tea and honey works well
No milk is used during attack, only fruit juice or alfalfa mint tea and honey

ARTHRITIS
Definition: any inflammatory or degenerative condition of a single joint or joints.

There are three major kinds of arthritis:

1.   Rheumatoid is the most serious type, since it can lead to crippling. It is a disease of the peripheral joints, but can also affect the lungs, blood vessels, the skin, spleen, and muscles, including the heart muscle. The early signs are usually fatigue, weight loss, muscular aches, stiffness in the joints, pain, a feeling of warmth in certain areas, and usually swelling. It comes on in acute stages of severe pain, swelling, and inflamation.

2.   Osteoarthritis causes a gradual degeneration of the joints. This type is often called the wear-and-tear disease, generally affecting people in later life. It is not generally inflammatory, nor does it usually cause general illness or affect parts of the body other than the joints. Often there is great pain. The pain can be a disabling and constant problem, especially in the knees and hips. Overweight and lack of muscle tone, create added burdens on the joints. It takes muscle to hold bones in place. Merely to rest or take pain pills does not remove the cause of the problem.

3.   Ankylosing spondylitis directly affects the spine, and often begins in the teens or twenties. It becomes a chronic inflamation of the spine.

NATURAL TECHNIQUE

The adrenocorticosteroids-related cortisone compounds have been used with some success for rheumatoid arthritis, because it has usually been brought about by adrenal exhaustion where insufficient cortin hormone has been produced. When cortisone was discovered, it was found to be helpful for this type of arthritis. Rheumatoid arthritis is not a gradually degenerative disease, but rather a sudden manifestation as a result of a traumatic experience: death in the family, shock, accident, overstress in business, or family. A complete exhaustion of the adrenal glands is caused by not enough of the cortin hormone necessary to handle the stress.

Steroid therapy with the use of cortisone, could have been an important advance in medial science, had it not been manufactured synthetically. There have been many disastrous side-effects from the use of cortisone, and people with all types of arthritis, where the adrenal gland is not the cause, have demanded this drug, causing more complications, until the medical doctors have become discouraged with its use. It has been used in many cases of skin condition, probably because the skin disease is often related to adrenal insufficiency. Skin rash is actually a blessing, because if the person did not break out and release the toxic wastes, they would be in serious pain from arthritis. Man often brings about a worse condition by attempting to stop nature's eliminative processes. However, he could stop both the arthritis and the skin condition if he would change the diet.

To use nature's remedies would seem far more reasonable than cortisone, with its side effects. The herb that acts like a steroid cortisone is Licorice root. The synthetic cortisone drug has been made from the Mexican wild yam. It would seem that the logical method to follow would be: cleansing the waste from the body, increasing the body's ability to use food, and correcting the chemical balance by adding the Licorice root. This would allow the body to act as if it had created the hormone, thus increasing the ability to utilize starches and meats until such time as it would produce on its own these necessary hormones. Then by killing the parasites feeding upon the accumulated toxic mucus, a healing crisis would slough off the mucus. It has been my experience to watch the wonders of a healing crisis when parasites have been killed. Globs of mucus will pour forth from the body.

It has been found that anti-malarial compounds modify rheumatoidal arthritis. This brings me to the conclusion that there are parasites involved, possibly the tubercular bacillus, or the malarial parasite. The malarial parasite can be killed by the use of Black walnut powder. The tubercular bacillus can also be killed by Black walnut. This disease seems to affect women more than men, and even children can develop it.

Losing weight, staying off the affected joints, resting, exercising, or taking pain pills, would be treating the effect and not removing the cause. Muscle tone requires high amounts of potassium to maintain strength. Calcium, phosphorus, and vitamin D are required to prevent the deterioration of the bones. In addition, a sound hormone balance is needed to utilize the foods properly so as to prevent a toxic build-up.

The things suggested by today's method of treatment would be like driving a car without tires. When stress is one of the causes, overcoming stress by resting, is often an impossibility. We sometimes have a tiger by the tail and cannot let go. Stresses have increased with technology. To have a natural hormone which would act as if the body had produced it and sufficient nutrition to rebuild the body so that one could stand whatever stresses life had to offer, would be a much better solution to the problem.

When people have lived to such great age in the past, it does not seem reasonable to me that deterioration by the age of fifty should become, as it has in our society, an accepted hazard. During the past fifty years, we in the United States, have become a degenerate people, both physically and spiritually. At the same time, scientific technology has accelerated. How can we be expected to stand up to the stresses of life? We must learn to eat the foods necessary for well being.

Herb teas are a very weak substitute for whole or powdered herbs. Certain herb teas are excellent and useful as a start, where fasting is involved, or for use with babies, but for chronic disease in adults, they are ineffective. My feeling is, that we should be tender and careful, even in the process of elimination. Take it easy and slow; nature's way is not sudden and immediate, but a gradual healing process. We live in such a world of "instant this" and "instant that", that we somehow expect to take a pill for instant health. The interesting thing about herbs is that they can be used alone, or dozens of them may be used together, without side effects. Quite often, a better result is achieved by using many herbs that complement each other.

Nature is still, in the final analysis, kinder than we suppose. It will not take as many years to overcome the disease as it took to arrive at such a state of degeneration.

Certain herbs, such as celery, alfalfa, chaparral, and saffron, have a tendency to return the calcium which is locked in the joints, into a solution, and move it out. They appear, either to have the ability to neutralize these acids or to regulate the hormone balance. Whichever it is, it works. Calcification and infiltration are proof to me that the body has not been receiving sufficient calcium, potassium, magnesium, phosphorus, and vitamin D, for its use in maintaining sufficient tone to prevent calcification, nor sufficient adrenal hormone to correctly utilize these minerals. Certain cases of osteoporosis occur where the bones become hollow and insufficient. At times, this hollowing is caused by the tubercular bacillus, and we call it bone cancer. We may again draw a relationship. Nevertheless, there is not enough material to maintain the bone structure being utilized by the body. This again brings us to the conclusion that we may need herbs to kill the parasites, and food herbs to rebuild a fine, more solid structure.

The facts about parasites are hideous, but inescapable, and problems with them will continue to persist until we learn how to keep our bodies clean and free of the mucus and wastes upon which parasites feed.

Sugar, leaches the vitamin B complex and calcium, from normal use in the body, leaving the nervous system stressed. This stress, then requires additional cortin. It is a vicious circle. When the intake of concentrated food is stopped, and an herb such as licorice root is added, (which acts in the body like the cortin hormone, reducing the stress) there is an excellent starting place for the arthritic patient. By adding sufficient vitamin B complex and calcium, along with the correct amount of the minerals which make calcium usable in the body (phosphorus, magnesium, vitamin D, etc.), a calmer attitude can be achieved, thus reducing the stress factor.

Where carrot and celery juice are not available, the experiments with alfalfa have been remarkable. Alfalfa has 34.9% calcium, along with all the related minerals that make calcium assimilable. Some thirty or forty tablets of alfalfa are sometimes required to be equivalent to the raw carrot juice therapy. There can be another problem with the arthritic when in adrenal exhaustion, which problem compounds the illness. The problem is a colitis condition, resulting from the lack of hydrochloric acid, brought on because of the lack of cortin hormone.

Large amounts of potassium are required to maintain muscle strength in osteoarthritis. Calcium, phosphorus, and vitamin D are required to prevent the deterioration of the bones. It is always amusing to me, when medical science persists in the assumption that diet plays no role in either the cause or the cure.

In ankylosing spondylitis, it is essential to stop the intake of concentrated foods and increase natural calcium. Alfalfa is the best source, taken in amounts of as much as twenty to forty tablets or capsules daily, along with approximately two to four capsules of licorice root. Children under 12 half of the adult dose.

A mild food diet is essential to heal arthritis. Carrot juice and celery juice, raw, about a quart each day for two weeks, and then one pint daily, 2 carrot and 2 celery until the arthritis is gone.

All forms of arthritis respond to the raw juice treatment in a most positive way. When using raw carrot and celery juices, carrot juice supplies the essential assimilable calcium, and the celery supplies the magnesium and the sodium, which seem to draw the calcium deposits out of the joints, when taken in quantities of a quart a day, along with a mild food diet. With mild food diet alone, the error in body chemistry seems to regulate, unless the parasite involvement is too high. With the addition of the cortisone-type herb, licorice root, and either chaparral, black walnut, or herbal pumpkin formula, even the most stubborn arthritis will begin to change. Renewed strength and vigor returns and pain should subside within the first few weeks.

CYSTIC FIBROSIS

Definition and pathology: The probable cause of the disease begins, not with the child, but with the poor diet of the mother, who was eating too many mucus-forming, concentrated foods. There is also a weakness in the gland function, which is passed on to the child. There is a possibility of damage to the neck, causing the choroid plexus gland to malfunction. This is the gland which regulates the secretion of the cerebrospinal fluid. This fluid must be maintained at a certain pressure level. When it is not correct in its functions, it has an effect on the medulla of the brain. The medulla regulates and controls the respiratory centers, the salivation, the heart, vomiting, sneezing, sweating, and swallowing. Damage to the choroid plexus could be the cause of the accumulation of toxic waste or could be the reason this waste cannot be readily expelled from the body. Then again, the accumulation of mucus from incorrect eating could cause the choroid plexus to be sluggish in its regulatory function. Either way, the result is still an accumulation of mucus, which is not easily removed from the body.

To be led along to the best answers, even for a disease considered terminal, is an interesting and rewarding quest, if it is approached with courage and faith. The most important thing in the final analysis, is not to escape death forever - no one is able to do that, but rather to find the best answers possible under a given circumstance. The final score will still add up, not to the winning or losing, but how well we played the game. How much pain and discomfort did we avoid, and how much health did we enjoy? There is always a better way to do something; it is just a matter of finding out what is the best way. There is also a reason that we need to go through trials. The best way to seek, is cheerfully, hopefully, and with the faith that you will find the answer.

NATURAL TECHNIQUE

A narcotic alkaloid, as suggested by medical doctors, in a disease of heavy mucus involvement, would cause the body to alkalize quickly. Continuous use of a narcotic to alkalize, allows the person to go on eating mucus-forming foods. The danger of continuous use, lies in possible addiction and also in the body becoming too alkaline - to the point where the body becomes devoid of minerals - as in alkaline soil. Alkalizing the body is nature's way to heal, and to be on the alkaline side is the best way to health, provided the body is maintaining the minerals it needs. A diet heavy in concentrated foods - starches, meats, and sugars - never provides enough mineral. When one drug is used to kill germs living on the refuse of such a diet (mucus), and another narcotic drug is used to alkalize, the results can be readily seen.

Cystic fibrosis is generally treated in this manner, creating not only side effects, but great dangers in taking the drugs. From my observation of natural healing methods, may I present an alternative solution to bring about as helpful a result as possible.

The herb which acts on the medulla and choroid plexus, is lady slipper. This wonderful herb, is one of the most expensive botanicals on the market. It is a relaxant herb, antispasmodic, nervine, and tonic, but acts primarily on the medulla, helping to regulate breathing, sweating, saliva, and heart functions. It is also called "moccasin flower". The plant grows in moist woodlands in many parts of Europe, Asia, and America. The blossoms have a sac-like lip shaped like a moccasin or slipper.

Change in diet is uppermost in cystic fibrosis. There is no way healing can take place without a change to the mild food diet. A formula for cleansing, as well as being nutritional, using some well established herbs in formula, will be most helpful.

Formula: Approx. 3 capsules daily for children, 6 capsules daily for adults
Lady slipper: 2 parts
Slippery elm: 1 part
Mullein: 1 part
Marshmallow: 1 part
Licorice root: 1 part
Poke root: 2 part

Mandrake: 2 part
Lobelia: 1/4 part
Cayenne: 1/4 part

Lady slipper: antispasmodic, nervine, and tonic, acts on the medulla and choroid plexus, which has to do with the heart, respiratory system, swallowing, saliva, and vomiting. The medulla and the choroid plexus, control all the exocrine glands. This is the major herb in this formula. Lady slipper may be used to act as a hormone when needed. The way to determine if more is needed, is when the congestion condition continues.

Slippery Elm: has a greater ability to remove mucus than any other herb and is very nutritious. Its demulcent capabilities are greater than most herbs, and it is capable of removing inflammation rapidly.

Comfrey: loosens mucus, soothes, stops bleeding or strong hemorrhaging and heals the lungs.

Alfalfa: is used in this formula for its nutritious properties. Alfalfa is also the natural hormone for the pituitary gland. This gland is the major regulatory gland of the body. Where the endocrine glands are affected, the exocrine glands will also be involved.

Mullein: is the anodyne or pain killer and is antispasmodic to stop spasms. It loosens mucus and moves it out of the system. It is strengthening to the lungs.

Marshmallow: is soothing for inflammation. It is also diuretic, and helps to move any fluid in the lung.

Lobelia: serves as a relaxant. Where breathing becomes hard there is great mental anguish, and Lobelia calms the soul. It also moves the obstruction which is often the cause of hard breathing.

Cayenne: for fever, and activates all other herbs to more useful purposes.

Licorice: gives added strength to the adrenal glands.

Poke Root: effective in acting on the liver. The liver can then function properly and aid in cleansing the body. It also has a flushing action on the entire body which aids in expelling waste. When used in conjunction with Cayenne it acts as a catalyst to generate heat.

Mandrake: the laxative part of the formula, designed to flush out toxic wastes. It also kills cancer parasites and other parasites in the body and assists in moving obstructions.

This formula and a mild food diet of fruits, vegetables, and lots of Vitamin C will allow the waste to be easily moved out of the body. It would logically follow that when a person has such weaknesses, it would be essential to live on a good diet continually in order to maintain general health and often use cleansing, maintaining herbs. This approach is a much more sensible way to maintain life with cystic fibrosis than to take dangerous drugs.

HEART DISEASE

Definition: the most common factors of heart disease are rheumatic, hypertensive, atherosclerotic, or pulmonary where the blood is not completely pumped out with each heart contraction so that circulatory disturbances follow, with the final result being heart failure. Arteriosclerosis is hardening of the arteries or faulty metabolism of fatty substances (such as cholesterol) clogging the artery wall, causing it to lose its elasticity, followed by gradual narrowing of the artery resulting in increased blood pressure.

NATURAL TECHNIQUE

My thinking is in agreement with Pritikin. It is my opinion, that too much fat in the diet has a great deal to do with many conditions, especially heart disease. The body needs certain fatty acids, however, for growth and development, as well as to sustain life. But, these fatty acids should come from finer oils, such as are found in nuts, fruit skins, vegetables, and seeds. If a person lives on a mild food diet, excluding the other oils, such as meats, dairy products, eggs, etc., they automatically improve, and heart disease is no exception to this rule. It seems strange, that 85% of the doctors are not reading their journals enough to discover that their training in drugs for heart patients is obsolete; so they continue to treat with the same methods. When sixty million people, almost one out of every two adults, has high blood pressure, it could be considered to be epidemic.

New diet ideas are popping up all over. Dr. John M. Douglas, internist at Kaiser Permanent Medical Center in Los Angeles, advises eating up to two cups of uncooked sunflower seeds each day to replace fatty foods in the diet. The seeds are good substitutes for food containing cholesterol and thus they lower the cholesterol level in the body. Even if the consumption of fatty foods is not decreased, the sunflower seeds will help fight cholesterol; it just makes the job a bit more difficult. Sunflower seeds contain linoleic acid, and eating them will tend to cut down the risk of heart disease.

The sense of taste is being scrutinized by scientists to determine what causes high blood pressure. Those with high blood pressure often are found to consume high amounts of salt. Their theory is, which comes first, the high blood pressure or a high-salt diet? Some scientists have hypothesized that people with high blood pressure may be eating more salt because of a weakened ability to taste it.

The salt intake generally has increased because of all the salt preservatives in packaged food, not to mention the salt drugs. It requires 5,000 mg. of potassium to compensate for 1 tsp. of salt. Living on the high concentrated food diet upon which the average American tries to survive, everything he consumes requires salt. No one would eat cake, cookies, pies, meats, candy, cereals, or breads, without salt, therefore potassium levels are extremely low in a high salt, concentrated food diet. Since potassium is the muscle toning mineral, and the heart is a muscle, it is no wonder that the incidence of heart failure is so high.

A mild food diet, excluding cooked oil, is essential to making a change in heart disease. No coffee, tea, alcohol, or tobacco, is allowed, if results are to be permanent. It has always been a great source of amazement to me to go out in the hall after one of my lectures and watch people light up their cigarettes, or at break time or lunch, during a health lecture, drink so much coffee. I feel it should go without saying, that anyone interested in good health would not use such drugs on a daily basis. Since that is not the case, it must be said.

NATURAL TECHNIQUE

Herbs: (adult doses listed; child's dose 9-14 years - 1/2 dose, 2-8 years - 1/3 dose)

A good cleansing herbal formula such as CD or CS, along with psyllium, is always a good place to begin. Use approx. 4-6 capsules of the cleansing formula. Psyllium powder or flakes, approx. 1-2 Tbs. Taken in water at the same time. Bedtime is usually the best time to take this.

Cayenne is used for all heart problems except hypertension. It is not used for hypertension, because it is the highest stimulant in the herb kingdom. Therefore, to bring hypertension down, the nervine relaxant herbs are used, such as lobelia, catnip, valerian, scullcap, lady slipper, hawthorn, and red clover. Cayenne is also used at the onset of a heart attack and will relieve it immediately - take 1 tsp. in a cup of hot water. Cayenne is wonderful when used for low grade fevers (rheumatic fever) and prostrating diseases. Cayenne increases power or acts as a catalyst for all other agents used. This is the reason it can be found in so many herbal formulas. Cayenne is used in all heart disease, except hypertension, with great success.

Hawthorn is used for any and all heart problems, even hypertension, and was used by every medical doctor up until about 1925, when botanicals were "out" and drugs became the "in" thing. Hawthorn seems to have a way of healing, repairing, soothing, and generally helping the heart in all respects.

Vitamins: (adult doses listed; child's dose 9-14 years - 1/2 dose, 2-8 years - 1/3 dose)

Vitamin E has been the standby vitamin in natural healing, even before Dr. Evan and Wilfred Shute wrote, Your Heart and Vitamin E. Even though their work gave credence to all that was believed in the health industry, it has still struggled for existence among their colleagues of the medical world. The results are clear and excellent, and those who have used vitamin E, especially for angina pain, swear by it. Use approx. 600 - 800 IU daily; rheumatic heart approx. 600 IU for 3-4 weeks, then increase to 800 IU for adults. High blood pressure requires careful supervision. Results are slow in the beginning, with eventual great value.

Vitamin B complex and Calcium (either lactate or preferably gluconate) used equally, become the best tranquilizer there is for hypertension, without side effects. This combination should be taken over and above the daily vitamin and mineral. It can be used in small amounts of approx. two calcium and two B complex and up to as many as six of each. Hyperactive children or nervous children, respond well to B complex and calcium for a calming effect.

Never eat food after 4:00 or 5:00 at night
An early supper should be light, mostly fruit. The main meal, consisting of vegetables, salads, sprouted grain, and sprouted grain breads, should be eaten at noon.
Drink lots of raw vegetable juices throughout the day.
A good multi-vitamin and mineral compound should be used on a daily basis.

Sometimes, inflamation will gather around the heart, causing pain. This condition should be treated the same as for a cold.

High blood pressure can sometimes be caused by calcium deposits around the heart. This can be removed in the same way calcium is removed from the joints in arthritis, or the arteries, by approx. one quart of celery juice daily for about 3 weeks.

For heart weakness, niacin is another good stimulant, especially where fibrillation or palpitations begin to occur. Niacin seems to give strength to rhythm, not speed, to a weak pulse. Usually, approx. 100 mg. a day will be sufficient.

KIDNEY DISEASE

Symptoms: lassitude (exhaustion), decreased mental ability, fatigue, muscular cramps, digestive disorders, muscle twitches, distorted sensory and motor abilities, malnutrition, and tissue wasting. The skin is discolored and urea sweat causes a uremic frost on the skin, often with itching that is very uncomfortable. Hypertension is also present most of the time.

If we understand the great responsibility of the kidneys, as one of the major organs of elimination, and correct body metabolism, all of the drug poisons and poor diet accepted by medical science borders on insanity, as far as the kidneys are concerned.

There are herbs that act on the kidneys in a diuretic manner to draw fluid. There are herbs that are soothing for inflammation, and there are herbs that rebuild and strengthen.

In the first place, when the kidneys are not functioning well, to the point of neuromuscular excitability (twitching muscles), or cardiac arrhythmias, etc., it is important to use laxative herbs to flush the waste out through the bowel and let the kidneys rest. A lot of diuretic herbs would not do in this case. There are herbs like juniper and goldenseal root, however, that are somewhat diuretic, but they also have the ability to be both antibiotic as well as healing to the kidneys. Bleeding from the bladder or severe kidney infection can be helped in a short period of time, with these wonderful herbs. Adult dose; approx, 2 capsules of juniper and 1 capsule of goldenseal root, children take 1/2 the dosage.

Pain in the kidneys can be relieved within a few minutes after chewing a few juniper berries. Juniper may also be taken in a powder or oil form. I have seen kidney infections of long standing, a year or

88

more, healed in just a few days, from taking juniper oil, using only 4-5 "o" size capsules a day for adults and 1/2 this amount for children.

When laxatives are used for extended periods, which are often necessary until the kidneys have a chance to rebuild with correct diet and herbs, potassium gluconate should be added to maintain muscular tone. Approx. 4-9 capsules daily for adults and 1/2 this amount for children.

The skin should also be activated to the utmost, so as to assist the kidneys to heal; brushing, loofah, massage, fresh air, sun baths, and sauna or steam baths are helpful. The intake of salt should be stopped or at least cut down to extremely small amounts. Sodium chloride (salt is a rock chemical and its molecular structure is too large to pass through the human body, even in a liquid state), is difficult to assimilate without causing irritation and over-work of the kidneys. The body needs natural sodium, and it is interesting that when high sodium food is used with kidney problems, such as straight celery juice, it draws off instead of causing it to retain fluid the way salt does. If you were to go on a scale from one to one hundred, celery would be approx. 65% sodium. Celery juice is one of the best treatments to use for fluid retention, approx. a quart a day, or a glass of distilled water with approx. 2 Tbs. of chlorophyll, taken 4-5 times daily, runs a very good second choice to pull off fluid.

NATURAL TECHNIQUE

Mild food is necessary for complete healing. No salt should be allowed in the diet. Dehydrated vegetable powders can be purchase as salt substitutes. Most mild food does not require salt the way concentrated food does. If people could learn to use condiment herbs to make food taste like gourmet meals, they would not need all the salt they use.

If cayenne and some other condiments are cooked, they become an irritant to the kidneys. Only add them to cooked foods, along with the soft oil being used, after the food has cooled a little.

HERBS HELPFUL FOR FAILING KIDNEYS

Laxative herbs:
  Senna
  Cascara sagrada
Soothing herbs:
  Comfrey
  Slippery elm
  Marshmallow
  Psyllium
  Solomon's seal
Healing, strengthening herbs:
  Alfalfa
  All-heal
  Barberry
  Chamomile
Diuretic herbs:
  Dandelion
  Cornsilk
  Horsetail
Nephritis herbs:
  Cow herb
  Foxtail
  Ribwort
  Radish

People who develop kidney stones, are lacking in magnesium, and usually have a problem with calcium-magnesium balance.

Vitamins: (adult doses listed; child's dose 9-14 years - 1/2 dose, 2-8 years - 1/3 dose)
Vitamin C: Approx. 3,000-4,000 mg. daily
A good multi-vitamin and mineral
Additional calcium. Carrot calcium is very good and
  can be purchased.
Vegetable juices that can help overcome uric acid in the body are:
  Beet

Carrot
Spinach
Parsley

No alcohol, coffee, black tea, or drugs should be used where kidneys are not functioning well.

KIDNEY INFECTION

(adult doses listed; child's dose 9-14 years - 1/2 dose, 2-8 years - 1/3 dose)
Enema
Vitamin C: 4,000-5,000 mg. daily
Goldenseal root: 4-6 "oo" size capsules daily
Juniper Oil: 4-6 "o" size capsule daily
Potassium gluconate: (will take off fluid) 4-5 99 mg. tablets
Kidney herbs: (used separately or in a formula)
Cornsilk - diuretic and healing
Juniper berries - diuretic and excellent
Dandelion - diuretic and excellent
Alfalfa - diuretic and also nourishing

KIDNEY STONE

(adult doses listed; child's dose 9-14 years - 1/2 dose, 2-8 years - 1/3 dose)
Stop all eating
Juice of one lemon straight, every time pain comes on, continue about every 15 minutes until stones are dissolved. It is not usually necessary to take lemon juice longer than 12-14 hours.
Goldenseal root: approx. 3-4 capsules daily
Hot enema when pain has subsided
Lobelia tea can be used as a relaxant

Kidney stones will dissolve with lemon, like water on rock salt, melting away the sharp edges. These sharp edges cut like glass on their way through, causing swelling and intense pain. With a kidney stone, the pain can be as severe as a difficult delivery of a baby. (A man who has passed a kidney stone knows what a difficult birth can be like.) The taking of lemon juice is such an easy thing, and works so well, it is hard for me to understand why medical science has not discovered so simple a remedy.

If the stomach has been irritated and become sore after stones have been dissolved, slippery elm, approx. 2 capsules before each meal, will overcome soreness.

MUSCULAR DYSTROPHY

Definition and pathology: Muscular Dystrophy is a disease where the muscles waste and atrophy. As the disease proceeds, virtually all muscles of the body become involved, leading to a terminal condition. Final complications are usually related to serious involvement with respiratory muscles.

There is no known medicine for the disease, but we know in the natural health field, that this disease responds favorably to corrective diet and herbs. We know further that the disease can be arrested, and by continued care, with diet and useful herbs, life can be extended many years. A good example of this is my Aunt Loree Griffin who tells her own story here:

My background was completely devoid of health teachings. Major childhood diseases struck me in severe forms – whooping cough, scarlet fever, diphtheria, even a burst appendix when I was ten years old. I enjoyed physical activity but at a young age found it difficult to keep up with friends.

I married and gave birth to three children after which my health problems increased, and I was told that I had "creeping paralysis". I spent years and thousands of dollars going to medical specialists of various types – some in distant cities – the diagnosis was always the same: hopeless, no known cure. Along the way, I endured numerous surgeries that were considered "emergencies" – I felt that every internal organ that I could live without had been removed.

Many times I would ask the doctors if there was anything I could do to improve my condition and help myself. What about nutrition and natural vitamins which I had read about. I was told that what I ate made no difference to my condition and vitamins would help not at all.

After I underwent a complete hysterectomy at age thirty-five the doctor said I would benefit if a visiting nurse gave me a hormone and vitamin shots – which I consented to, as I was physically unable to go to the doctor's office. After three years of such medication every week, I felt I was at the end of the line. I soon learned that "incurable muscular dystrophy" was the new name given for my affliction. I was confined to bed most of every day.

A neighbor told me of a – Dr. Bernard – was going to be in Sacramento for several days, and I should try to see him. My faith was weak, but in desperation I made the appointment. That began the change in my life when I was past middle age. Dr. Jensen asked me no questions. As he looked sharply at me and my eyes, he marked a diagnostic chart and wrote down a list of herbs and natural foods which I should have.

My wonderful husband, Lee, was always most cooperative and went to the health food store and obtained the items. Thus began the long and difficult task of changing nutritional habits of half a – it wasn't – the results began to show before long. I used various herbs in teas which began to balance my acid system, and added natural vitamins.

I was overjoyed when my niece, LaDean Griffin, published her years of research in books (Is Any Sick

Among You? and No Side Effects) for they have proved an invaluable reference for me. I began experimenting with her formulas and received marked benefit. Everyone needs all of them at some time for varied conditions. I appreciate the way she ties in the temporal aspect of the use of herbs with the spiritual. They are truly a food and medicine from the Lord. My belief is that our Heavenly Father has given us all we need to this earth for health and happiness and it is up to us to seek out what is best for us as individuals and utilize it accordingly. Of course that includes accepting knowledge of truth and using self-discipline and willpower to apply the principles to our lives.

I am now in my seventieth year and could never have made it without this help, for which I am truly grateful. I have continued my health program though the years, and with the help of the Lord have been able to meet the vicissitudes of life with faith and a strong spirit. I am sure my life has specifically been prolonged so that through my experiences, my posterity might benefit. I tell my family that when I leave this mortality it will be because my work here is finished and I will be ready for eternity.

Loree A. Griffin

The problem with muscular dystrophy is that it cannot be detected clinically until 50% of the cytocytes for muscular tissue cells are affected. Parents need to be more aware of a child's body tone and how it should be, to indicate health. Today, however, children are so flabby because of the poor diets of their parents and the kinds of junk foods they are raised on, that the average parents do not know the difference until it is too late and the disease is well developed. If a new understanding of an old truth could somehow be established, many people, in their youth, could be spared the misery of diseases like muscular dystrophy. The way to spare a flabby child such a fate is to change his diet to more fruits and vegetables and take away concentrated foods, such as meats, starches and sugars. We know this because terminal muscular dystrophy cases are able to survive on such a regimen. Why does it work? Potassium is the major muscle-toning mineral and can be found in large amounts in such things as mutton and beef, but anytime the body is already weak and sickly, such foods become almost a poison, causing more strain on glands and digestive organs as they make such potassium available to use in the body.

With fruits and vegetables, nuts and seeds, the glands and organs do not have to overwork to use readily available potassium, as well as all other related minerals for the strength and vigor. A person who is weak, generally builds toxic waste and more sickness on heavy concentrated foods faster than a person with normal health. He therefore responds to the foods he can use, assimilate, and digest without leaving a toxic residue. Fruits and vegetables are such foods. Besides being the best source of potassium, vegetables and fruits act like a broom, maintaining not only the peristaltic action of the colon with the bulk but keeping any toxic waste from building up in tissues or bowel. Concentrated foods have a tendency to become sludgy, constipating and sticky in the bowel, thereby causing a toxic condition because the ability to eliminate waste is inhibited. Certain herbs are helpful in Muscular Dystrophy simply because they act to clean out the already accumulated waste, as well as to add necessary vitamins and minerals to a diet probably lacking in proper nutrients. Insufficient potassium results in other symptoms besides flabby, weak muscles such as the following:

low blood sugar
paralysis
water retention
listlessness
fatigue
general constipation
pulse weak, slow, or irregular
heart attack or degeneration of heart muscle
swollen testicles or ovaries
foggy thinking
prolapses of colon
swollen ankles
dry throat

kidney damage
bitter taste in mouth

Loss of body potassium occurs from taking drugs, specifically cortisone, aspirin, ACTH, diuretic water pills and even too much salt in the diet. We note that concentrated foods required too much salt in order to be palatable. For example, you would not eat cake, cookies, bread or cereal without salt: neither would you eat meat. Because Americans eat such a high concentrate food diet, they consume at least 1 to 5 teaspoons of salt daily. It takes 5,000 mg of potassium to compensate for 1 teaspoon of salt in the diet. When people eat that much concentrated food, they are too full to eat the necessary fruits and vegetables to make up the deficit. Another cause of potassium loss is stress. Sugar in the diet causes stress because it leaches the Vitamin B and Calcium from the body, leaving the nervous system undernourished. We can therefore see why such foods are not desirable with muscular dystrophy for potassium purposes, but will also contribute to the lack of potassium. Another probable relationship is that the body requires a correct balance of sodium and potassium to activate nerve response.

NATURAL TECHNIQUE

Corrective diet is essential in helping diseases of muscles. Certain vitamins and mineral are of utmost importance, as follows:

Vitamin B1: for general strength
Vitamin B12:   (if any meat is used) for cell longevity, healthy nervous system and correct protein and carbohydrate metabolism.
Biotin: for cell growth, Vitamin B utilization, and to stop muscular pain.
Niacin: increases hormone production, reduces cholesterol levels, increases circulation, stimulates hydrochloric acid production and increases muscle strength.
Pantothenic acid: increases ability to form antibodies, stops muscle cramps.

Foods high in B
    Asparagus
    Beets
    Brussel sprouts
    Carrots
    Cauliflower
    Lettuce
    Bananas
    Figs
    Strawberries
    Watermelon

Magnesium - necessary for the utilization of calcium as well as Vitamin C.
    Foods high in magnesium:
    Watercress
    Leeks
    Tomatoes
    Leaf lettuce
    Parsnips

Phosphorus: necessary for utilization of Calcium, Vitamins A and D, iron and manganese: Regulates heart muscle contraction and cell growth.

    Foods high in Phosphorus:
    Artichokes
    Kale
    Dates

Potassium: regulates heart beat, growth and muscle contraction; is a tranquilizer for the nerves. The lack of potassium results in muscle damage, weak reflexes, nervousness, irregular heart beat and general lack of muscle tone, flabby weak muscles.

    Foods high in Potassium:
    All fruits
    All vegetables

Copper: needed for red blood production and general healing processes. Without copper, there is general body weakness, but only trace amounts are necessary. It is found in fruits and vegetables.

Manganese: the enzyme activator assisting with growth. The lack of manganese results in muscle coordination failure.

Foods high in Manganese:
    Turnips
    Corn
    Almonds
    Brazil nuts

Herbal Formula for Muscular Dystrophy: Approx. 4-5 capsules daily. (adult doses listed; child's dose 9-14 years - 1/2 dose, 2-8 years - 1/3 dose)

    Kelp - 1/4 part
    Mullein - 2 part
    Alfalfa - 1 part
    Parsley - 1/8 part
    Raspberry - 1/4 part
    Licorice Root - 1 part
    Burdock Root - 1/4 part
    Yellow Dock - 1/8 part
    Mandrake - 1/4 part
    Comfrey - 1/8 part
    Lady slipper - 1/4 part

Kelp: a good source of B12 and E, niacin and manganese and iodine. Iodine is helpful in this formula for physical and mental development.

Mullein: for magnesium and potassium

Alfalfa: one of our best vitamin and mineral – 34.9% calcium with sufficient D, phosphorus and magnesium to make calcium usable in the body. High in potassium, chlorine, sodium and silicon has Vitamin E, A, B12, and even B6. One of our most effective vitamin herbs. Alfalfa will stop muscle spasms and cramps within minutes.

Parsley: is a good source of copper.

Raspberry: for B1 – source of E.

Licorice: is not only a good phosphorus source, but gives strength to the adrenal glands.

Burdock root: contains B3, niacin and Vitamin C. Burdock root is a helpful addition to this formula but it also is one of the best blood purifiers. It keeps waste moving out of a weak body. Where there is weak muscle structure and general weakness, toxic waste is more rapidly accumulated. Increases the flow of urine.

Yellow Dock: tones the entire body and is a powerful tonic. Is used for its excellent ability to purify the blood.

Mandrake: laxative, regulator of the liver and bowels. Acts thoroughly on the lymphatic system to expel waste that would otherwise accumulate when there is muscle weakness.

Comfrey: a powerful herb for inflammation and general weakness.

Lady Slipper: the nervine herb used in this formula because it is so useful where any brain damage may be part of a muscular problem. Lady Slipper also relieves pain which may be associated with muscular problems.

After having watched Aunt Loree maintain her life for the all of the 27 years I have known her, I know she is a living witness to the things she had adhered to. She is a beautiful lady. It is my prayer along with hers, that the things she has learned will bless her posterity. She celebrated her ninetieth birthday, August 1999.

DIABETES

Definition: The common theory today concerning diabetes is that it is a metabolic disorder where insulin deficiency causes the body to be unable to metabolize glucose adequately, thereby forcing the body to derive its major source of energy from the metabolism of lipids, particularly the fatty acids. It has been found, however, that an excessive amount of Ketone bodies (acetoacetic acid, beta hydroxybutyric acid, and acetone these are the end products of fat metabolism) are then produced.

Pathology: With this acidosis stage the excess acid causes the kidneys to spill off important potassium and sodium. When this occurs, the cardinal metabolic manifestations of diabetes begin to arise: hyperglycemia, glycosuria (sugar in the urine), and ketosis (incomplete combustion of fatty acids), often followed by ketoacidosis (acidemia).   With these errors established, the ramifications of the loss of glucose energy or usable glucose seems to fan out into wider circles, such as the inability to use proteins. At this point virtually all of the endocrine glands can be affected, principally the pituitary and adrenal glands.

There have been many theories propounded regarding the reason for the diabetic becoming diabetic and how the mechanism has a slow response when ingesting sugar. Does the problem lie in the gland's inability to empty the bowel form of insulin? Danowski wrote his theories in 1964; Luft in 1968; Antoniades and his associates in 1962; Owen and Lilley in 1961; Leibel and Wrenshall in1964 wrote on the connection of diabetes and the pituitary; Benson and Yallow wrote in 1965; Larsson in 1967. But with all these many opinions and bits and pieces of both theory and proven facts, an understanding of diabetes remains incomplete, and the frustration over the search for insulin inhibitors has led to serious concern.

The fact still remains that there is a great deal of unknown facts about – much evidence that it takes a great deal of courage to place confidence in medical control. There are so many related factors involved that daily changes and unique physiologies would require a continual vigil of day and night baby-sitting to be able to expect perfect help form the doctor. If a person were to go into a sudden coma from what seemed to be the physician's negligence, a cost of several thousand dollars would be required to regulate it again. Could the patient be sure that it would never happen again? Certainly he could not, because the disease itself is impossible to stabilize permanently due to so many variables.

There are four main stages to diabetes:

1. Pre-Diabetes

Manifestation of certain diabetic symptoms before any abnormal glucose tolerance tests of carbohydrate metabolism. Usually suspected where there is strong hereditary predisposition to diabetes.

2. Latent Chemical Diabetes

Under stress, glucose tolerance tests are abnormal. In the absence of stress the test is normal, such as during pregnancy.

3. Chemical Diabetes or Latent Diabetes

Patient always show abnormal glucose slightly elevated and especially during stress. Needs only particular care during stress infractions or pregnancy.

4. Overt or Manifest Diabetes

Some people may start into manifest diabetes and shift back and forth. Sometimes obesity can have an effect on this. Excess body weight apparently cause an increase of up to three or four times the production of insulin. This increase probably stems from the increased need for disposition of insulin in the body fat. Weight loss can often convert the diabetic back to latent diabetes. Other factors may lead to the onset of the disease, such as hyperthyroidism or diabetes insipidus caused by the pituitary gland. The therapeutic administration of steroids often is a triggering influence. Sometimes infections can be the beginning factor. Obviously, then, diabetes depends on more than hereditary traits alone.

Pancreatic diabetes ensues when permanent damage has occurred because of surgical removal of Parts of the Body Essential For: the pancreas, performed to remove tumors. This type can also develop due to sever pancreatitis (inflammation of the pancreas), causing permanent damage to the islets of Langerhans.

The word glycosuria means sugar spilled off in the urine. Glycosuria can also be seen in severe emotional stress, hypothalamic or brainstem injury, hepatic disease or an abnormally low renal threshold. This would appear sometimes to indicate diabetes where glucose levels are really normal.

Hyperglycemia is defined as: Hyper-insulinism where the body calls on an excessive amount of insulin to handle the sugar and starch intake. Over-insulinising then causes a self-inflicted insulin form of shock, then dropping into low blood sugar.

Prolonged periods of hyperglycemia will eventually be the cause of diabetes, for the constant call for insulin exhausts the pancreas' ability to produce. It is believed by some that inflammation in the pancreas is the initial cause of this over-insulinising reaction.

Surgery of the pancreas for tumors is a dangerous operative procedure, depending on the site and extent of the tumor. The prognosis for a patient with cancer on the main body of the pancreas is poor. The only time it is logical to carry out resection, according to the Canadian Journal of Surgery, is when the groove behind the neck of the pancreas in which the portal vein lies has not been invaded by the tumor.

The results of pancreas surgeries for carcinoma, Royal Melbourne Hospital in 1980 reports, after palliative bypass showed a mean survival or only 6.7 months. The problems after surgery would not seem worth it to me.

The rapid decline in general condition after a laparotomy (incision through the abdominal walls) and death occurring in 75% with a maximum survival after the operation was only three months.

A survey was quoted to emphasize the poor prognosis of carcinoma of the pancreas where one of the patients were cured and where 90% of those operated on were dead within one year.

Many surgeries are performed for the purpose of clinical observations, and certainly doctors have discovered by such surgeries what not to do.

Retinopathy is one of a number of long-term complications of diabetes. Others include cataracts, lens and kidney problems. Certain tissues such as muscle and adipose tissue are sensitive to the effects of insulin, allowing glucose carried in the blood to be taken up so these tissues never exhibit any of the long term degenerative changes that take place in diabetes. Those that do deteriorate, on the other hand, are the ones which are insensitive to insulin and they are the tissues which bear the full brunt of raised blood sugar levels. With high blood sugar levels in these areas, the vitreous parts of the eye can hemorrhage, causing the retina to detach. Scientist have learned how to re-attach the retina, but as long as the hemorrhages continue the diabetic will finally become blind.

Tests have shown that sucrose fed rats develop Retinopathy equally as fast as those fed on starch.

A great deal of work is being done today with dietary management of diabetes but for the most part the strict changes to mild food have not been determined. There remains much worry about protein or psychological problems associated with restricted diet. This discovery of stress relative to diabetes could include stress related to a restricted diet. A person must decide how well he or she wants to be and go from there. Some people would rather die than give up the foods they like.

Scientific studies note the Islet cells producing glucagon can cause the skin conditions relative to diabetes. No real answer as to how to deal with the condition has been forthcoming, however.

For more than half a century management of diabetes has been diet and insulin therapy, which has been totally unsuccessful and impossible to restore glucose homeostasis to normal. Transplants of the pancreas have even been done on dogs for a number of years but the final conclusions have been drawn that the cure for diabetes is not imminent.

Scientists are working on an artificial pancreas that can mimic the insulin-secreting beta cells. They are working on an analyzer to measure glucose which eventually can be implanted much like a cardiac pacemaker.

Definition and Pathology – Did you know that during 1964 each person in the United States consumed an average of 95 pounds of sugar? By 1979 it was estimated that level rose to 128 pounds per person. Much of this sugar is consumed in process foods, candies and table sugar. The demand for sweet tasting products and the desire of the food industry for longer shelf duration of products have combined to boost the use of sugar. Li and Schuhmann, in a study made in 1980, found sucrose and sucrose combinations present in 71 popular breakfast cereals, ranging in sugar content to as high as 55.6%.

The crime rate in the United States has been found to be related to the rise in sugar consumption, according to J.I. Rodale, in his article, "Does Sugar Make Criminals?" He related some startling experience, which I find very easy to believe, since I have observed the same things many times. One set of parent told me that their child would steal to get candy and after eating large amounts of candy would become violent to the point of threatening to kill his parents. When they removed sugar, meat and starch from his diet and fed him vegetables and fruits, he became a totally different sweet child.

Besides being nearly as addictive as alcohol, sugar can also create a comparable state of acidosis in the body. This condition can cause the person to become argumentative and angry like a drunk, or in some people, cause apparent joviality. Some people may even go into a stupor or become violent. Like alcohol, who can know if large amounts of sugar will produce a criminal or a teddy bear?

If you are saying, "Sugar gives me a lift and makes me happy, so I will continue to eat it, it may be well to consider its effects on your body and your life. Sugar leeches Vitamin B and calcium from the body, leaving the nervous system shattered. The more sugar one uses, the more nervous one becomes. The lack of calcium is reflected in hair loss, poor teeth and fingernails, and in osteoporosis, a condition in which bones become porous and soft. The lack of calcium causes brain problems such as senility and stupor, because calcium brings oxygen to the brain. Poor circulation, gland and hearing problems can result from the lack of calcium.

The ability to use sugar is directly related to the individual's hormone balance. Sugar, whether it be black strap, sorghum, raw, white or brown is still sucrose and requires sufficient insulin to be changed into glucose before it can be assimilated. When this change cannot be made effectively, sucrose is spilled out into the urine or absorbed into the blood. The body cannot use sucrose, and this condition causes acidosis, resulting in a coma. Insulin merely allows this change to be accurately accomplished. For the most part, older people who have become diabetic do so because they are junk food addicts, and have exhausted the pancreas trying to produce enough insulin to handle the constant flood of sugar. This causes a fault in the mechanism, which results in an overproduction of insulin, which causes the person to go into a form of insulin shock and then drops down into low blood sugar. Some people experience these highs and lows hourly and daily, making them very difficult people to live with. Often they are almost insane from their own vacillation.

The philosophy of those who treat diabetes has been to stay completely away from all sugars. However, honey and fruit are not sucrose, but are already glucose, and need no insulin to make the change to a usable form. To take a diabetic person completely away from fruit because it contains sugar would be to starve him of the natural glucose he needs to maintain life and energy levels. When a person is taking insulin, he feels (because of the protein theory) that he must eat starches and meats to maintain health. A good hormone balance is required to change starches and meats into the usable form, and when one gland, like the pancreas, is out of balance, other related glands do not always perform as they should. This causes the diabetic to easily develop an acidosis condition. The doctor will then give bicarbonate to neutralize the acid caused by inaccurate utilization of meats and starches, and then give needed glucose to maintain – the life of a diabetic! However, when a diabetic goes on a mild food diet of fruits, vegetables, nuts and seeds (which are mostly glucose), the acid begins to alkalize, causing the burden of the acidosis to be lessened. Until the body is completely alkaline and clean, natural herbal insulin is required. It is also necessary to discover whether there are parasites involved, and to rid the pancreas of them.

People who are ill and unable to take food in a normal way are often given a glucose solution directly into the blood, which would again tend to prove Professor Ehret's theory that it is grape sugar, not protein, that builds the body. We know that even glycogen (a polysaccharide animal starch) is derived in the body from glucose, especially found in the liver and muscles, and that another change takes place to change grape sugar into glycogen. This proves that it is grape sugar, not protein which maintains; and fats also must be changed into glucose before being used, with hormone stimulation the cause to bring it about. It is my conclusion once more that as Professor Ehret has stated, it is grape sugar or glucose which is fuel for the human body. This is the reason fruit is a superior food.

It is my opinion that hormones are essential to allow proper change of fats, proteins, complex sugars and starches into glucose. It is also my opinion that when insufficient hormones are secreted into the body from any or all glands, the body becomes toxic (which, of course, it can become due to wrong combination and non-nutritious toxin-forming foods), fats and undigested proteins and starches remain in the blood as cholesterol or hardened fat (overweight). In this sense, both starches and sugars are turned into fat. The opposite occurs in some cases of diabetes when sufficient insulin hormone to make the change from protein and starch and complex sugars to simple sugar or glucose are used. If natural simple sugars of fruit are used, it is easier on the already sick body; however, it is still necessary to have enough insulin hormone to affect the utilization of the glucose in maintaining the body until it becomes clean. When sugar spill off in the urine and is not used, the body will waste away.

With the exception of where there has been organic damage, the first thing to bring about a cure would be to remove the cause (the parasite), having sufficient insulin or the herb insulin to maintain the body until the glands begin to produce again.

It is with difficulty that the normal glucose sugar can be restored to correct levels even when using fruit sugars and honey. Fruit sugar and honey are already glucose and require no insulin to allow them to be used by the body, but the toxic condition of the diabetic coming in contact with natural glucose sugars cause fermentation, gas distress and acid stomach, so that the person becomes discouraged from eating fruits and slips back into bad habits of eating mucus-forming foods. This fermentation and acid can be relieved by the use of Saffron and Dandelion, both of which act on the liver and kidneys. Mucus-forming foods seem at first to be easier to tolerate. In the long run they only contribute to the disease. When a diabetic has reached the state of the disease that he can no longer tolerate proteins that he often changes over to fats for energy, thus resulting in acidosis. With the inability to efficiently use protein and eating more fats, it can be seen how the rapidly developing lipid plaques can form. The iris of the eyes shows the wasting body filled with toxic waste as the diabetic disease proceeds.

During this discussion of diabetes, we must talk about sugar. Glucose sugar (chemical formula $C6H12O6$) is about half as sweet as cane sugar. We call it dextrose or grape sugar. It is the sweetness we taste in fruit, seeds, leaves, flowers, honey and roots. Glucose is found in the bodies of men and animals (the cause of the sticky sweetness of blood). Glucose is a sugar which does not need to be digested. When taken into the body, molecules or particles of glucose pass directly through the walls of the small intestines, the place from which all nourishment is absorbed into the bloodstream. Glucose carried into the blood oxidizes to supply heat and energy to all of the body. Sugar turns into fats and to muscles. A pig does not get fat from being fed fats; he get fat from eating corn.

All other carbohydrates and all sugars of a complex nature must be broken down by digestion into this simple grape sugar or glucose before they can be utilized by the body. It has been proven that normally indigestible cellulose found in vegetables breaks down into glucose by intestinal bacterial action. In the normal person, glucose makes up to 0.1 percent of the blood. In the diabetic person, the amount of glucose in the blood is increased and is spilled off unused into the urine. Glucose is given directly into the veins when a person is unable to take food.

For the diabetic, the question may arise, "How is it possible to live on glucose sugar intravenous feedings?" When glucose is used, antibiotics are usually necessary after the first few days to stop infection, because the medical scientists do not realize that the moment a person goes into a fasting state, the body begins to eliminate waste, causing the acute infections that occur while taking only intravenous feedings. It has been assumed that the cause is a lack of protein, because as soon as protein is eaten, the elimination stops. When a person cannot take in protein, it is thought that the lack of protein causes the protein deterioration that accompanies an overwhelming elimination of toxic waste into the blood.

The diabetic needs to have insulin to utilize sucrose sugar and starches so as to make the change to simple glucose sugar. However, most diabetics can eat fruit or honey without insulin as long as starches are not eaten in the same meal. This is why they can take glucose in the veins, but here again the body will begin its fasting elimination. When the body arrives at a serious stage of elimination, the person often dies of pneumonia or other infection unless antibiotics are administered. As toxic waste moves into the blood, causing heavy obstruction to bodily functions, and when, in a weakened condition, the waste cannot be moved out, death usually follows. The body's protein begins its deterioration process as death proceeds in its course to end life. When this deterioration reaches a certain point, death occurs.

If the body were clean and free from waste it could continue for extended periods on glucose in the veins. There is another factor, however, indispensable after a while to strength, which is a part of the creating of fuel, heat and energy. The breakdown of bulk which causes combustion has a real part in the continuance of life, but it does not have to be protein bulk, adding only more toxic waste to the already sick body, unable to accurately make necessary changes. Does this give hope to the terminally diseased person? Yes, it does when it is understood.

There are some cases of diabetes where insulin in the blood is higher than non-diabetics, indicating to me that there is a failure of the mechanism binding insulin in the plasma. This in an observation in cases usually of a mature nature. This indicates to me also that the person had a hyperglycemic condition prior to the onset of diabetes, causing the constant over-demand for insulin, bringing on the insulin shock and resultant low blood sugar slump. In a fasting state most insulin remains bound to the substance part of the plasma. As soon as glucose is given, bound insulin disappears rapidly and unbound insulin increases, moving out in the blood to prepare for use. This should tell us that there is even a certain function connected to insulin affecting the use of glucose. As I see it, there are two definite parts: one to change sucrose and starch to glucose, and another to utilize glucose. In most cases it is only the first. In giving intravenous feeding, the insulin must be kept at a correct level and acid must be brought down to alkaline and also infection (elimination) must be kept down – a very complicated touch and go situation.

Now if there were herbs that could normalize all factors this would be a great advantage. The interesting thing about the insulin-type herbs is that this is exactly what they do: the same way Kelp works on either hypo- or hyper-thyroid.

In order to help the diabetic in a natural way we must first start by killing the parasites. This is followed by reducing tension and of course, taking herbs which act like insulin, allowing the body to use sucrose sugars. It is my opinion that natural herbs which act like insulin do much more than that; however it can be seen that the toxic residue of the disease is built up because of the body's inability to use fats and oils correctly as a result of sugar loss.

After watching the changes that occur in the iris as diabetes is healed, I am convinced that for the most part there are parasites involved both in causing the disease and because of the disease.

For example: When the child seems to develop diabetes early and suddenly, it is my opinion that the parasites, salmonella or trichinosis, usually begin growth in the small intestine and spread eventually through the entire body. They become deeply embedded and entirely fill the pancreatic gland, more particularly the islet of Langerhans. The adult trichinosis live about six weeks. During this life span, one female produces 1,500 larvae. These larvae are carried by the blood and become lodged in the capillaries of any organ or tissue of the body. They have been found in all organs of the body, even in the milk of the nursing mother, thereby being transmitted to the nursing child. Children and young people acquire these parasites from any or all of the sources: from the mother's milk, incorrect mucus diet, unclean surrounding, or bad chicken or pork. It is my opinion that this explains why very young children develop diabetes. It has been previously thought that it was hereditary, but not in the manner recognized. It has been my interesting observation that when these parasites are killed by using certain herbs, the accumulated mucus upon which they feed will be expelled during a healing crisis. The interesting thing which also occurs at this point is that the eye changes as the toxic waste is moved and parasites killed.

Parasites cannot take hold unless the body is overly encumbered with toxic waste due to incorrect diet or inherent weakness, such as slow metabolism, or low blood pressure. Neither can parasites or germs live on healthy, sound tissue. We do not have maggots in our sink or in our garbage cans because we keep them clean. The body is in a constant state of trying to return us to dust at the slightest provocation. Whenever there is waste matter which is not expelled from the body, it serves as food for parasites and germs. If the body were maintained at a sound and completely nourished state in which all body wastes were burned or expelled, there would be no need to fear the microbe nor his undesirable cousins.

Many people live in a half-decayed state and do not recognize it, other than to know that they do not feel well. Nature has already performed in their bodies a great deal of her work before the body is laid in the ground. With these parasites crying for more of the kind of foods they can thrive on, continually calling to the person in whose body they have taken up residence, it seems to the person that he cannot get enough candy, cake and goodie junk in general. His hunger for sweets in unbearable, so he promptly obeys the call of his now well-associated friends and gives them what they want, thus giving them food to grow upon and propagate their young. This cycle continues the diabetic state (if the parasites have invaded the pancreas sufficiently), fast approaching the beginning of a disease he will live with from then on, until it eventually becomes his executioner.

When some people, especially children, suddenly become diabetic, (in the author's opinion) it is because parasites have invaded the islets of Langerhans and have retarded and then stopped insulin production. When the parasites are removed by herbs such as Pumpkin seed or Black Walnut, normal insulin production will be resumed, if there has been no permanent damage to the glands.

Studies made by Siperstein, 1964, explain that elevated levels of plasma glycoprotein may contribute to the development of hyaline membranes. It is my opinion that this is the effect rather than the contributing cause. The cause is the individual's reaction to stress. It has been found that substantial doses of Vitamin B Complex and Calcium Gluconate change the nerve rings on the iris of the eye, indication that the nervous system is then more relaxed. However, some people require more relaxation of the nervous system than others because of the way that they react to stress. Some people live in a self-made torture chamber of fear and worry and would not seem to be happy in any other state. Consequently, their stress levels are always higher.

The nervine herbs are more helpful, either in combination or by themselves. Studies of relaxant or sedating drugs would prove to anyone the danger of a diabetic person taking such drugs. It take s a good healthy body to take either pain-killing drugs or relaxants. It requires sound liver and kidney response, and often the diabetic has neither. Therefore, it seems logical to use vitamins and herbs instead to help relieve such nervous tension. Medical science has presented their many ideas about diabetes with little agreement on how or why insulin works. The main thing they write about is how to die of this disease. It seems to me to be my duty to give another answer or alternative to help the diabetic who wishes to try natural methods.

It is recognized that the hormone insulin, when produced by the body, is a protein molecule. By the same method, a mother producing milk for her baby, when living on nothing but fruit can produce a protein milk. A richer protein milk is not produced by eating meat and in most cases, I would say, is not as rich. It is interesting to note that a diabetic, or any person who has a hormone imbalance; adrenal, thyroid, or pituitary, has the inability to digest meat at all in the later stages of disease.

There are so many opinions on the subject, and since few of them agree, except in the need for insulin and the value of insulin control; let me here give my opinion of the subject relative to herbs and natural foods versus drugs and accepted orthodox treatments. Some in the medical worlds are so indoctrinated with drug theory that they dare not look at anything else.

It is interesting to observe that Goldenseal and Juniper, which can take the place of insulin in a natural herb form, are both diuretics, which would seem inconsistent for diabetes, where the main symptom would be glycosuria. Nevertheless, these herbs not only have an action similar to insulin, but have a healing ability to the entire body. Juniper is one of the finest herbs available for healing and restoring the kidneys. This action is so immediate that the ache of kidney pain can be removed within minutes after chewing a few of the berries. Goldenseal can stop a bleeding bladder infection overnight or within a few hours. (This makes a useful remedy, since the kidney is one of the most frequently and severely affected organs in diabetes.) These two remarkable herbs have also a wonderful antibiotic ability. Goldenseal used on a diabetic sore will heal when nothing else will.

We should mention also the impact of diabetes on the unborn child. Stillbirths are common among diabetic mothers. If the child is born alive, it will usually be much larger than normal because of edema and has a poor chance of survival. Since research has not been done to know why Goldenseal and Juniper work as insulin, no one knows how or why they work, but it may be interesting to note that Goldenseal reduces internal swelling and can stop internal bleeding immediately.

Diabetics also often develop an iron anemia. The total quantity of iron in the body should be 4 to 5 grams in an adult. American diets contain 10 to 15 mgs. a day and only about 10 percent is absorbed. Often iron is not absorbed because of an incorrect diet. Iron is destroyed by narcotic drugs and coffee. There are many herbs high in iron. Alfalfa is 1.30% iron, which is high for a trace mineral. Meadow Sweet, Mullein, Parsley, Red Raspberry, Silverweed, Stinging Nettle, Strawberry Leaves, Watercress and Yellow Dock are some of the high iron herbs.

In later stages of diabetes disease the pancreas develops fibrosis while the liver develops cirrhosis. It becomes very dangerous therefore, for a diabetic to take sedative or relaxant drugs, since the liver can no longer detoxify the drugs. Medical science has supposedly come to the rescue with fanfare, the discoveries being knighted and given the Nobel Prize. To an extent, they have prolonged the patient's life, provided his is a very methodical and remarkably organized individual. He must br accurate in his analysis of each symptom as it occurs and take exactly the amount of insulin required.

F. G. Banting and C. H. Best have discovered that the body would accept the hormone (as it was named) of an animal and use it as if the person himself had produced it. At the time there was no exact knowledge on the principle of the chemical nature of internal secretions. It was a great discovery, and many discoveries have been added since this doorway of new knowledge has been opened to our view: cortisone, thyroid, ACTH, estrogen and testosterone. However, nothing for the diabetic was discovered to effect a cure, rather a promise of continued life as long as insulin is available to the user. Continual shots and a careful diet: this would be his status for the rest of his life.

One main advantage to the use of Goldenseal as opposed to insulin is that is stops internal bleeding. In later stages of diabetes the vitreous part of the eye begins to hemorrhage, causing the retina to detach with resultant blind spots and eventual complete blindness. By using Goldenseal this does no happen, nor do the running sores of later stages occur – the plague of the diabetic. Goldenseal must be used in the same methodical way as insulin in order to avoid coma. If Goldenseal is added to regular insulin shots, shock can be the result. Lowering the regular intake of insulin and using Goldenseal in increased amounts as insulin is lowered, is the way people have gotten off insulin.

Linda Clark says in her book, Color Therapy, that radiating the livers of diabetics with orange light reduces daily intake of insulin from 145 to 25 units. Medical science has learned to use light color therapy on jaundiced babies with excellent results. Perhaps they will soon see the value of light color therapy for the diabetic as well as the use of herbs and a mild food diet.

Of all people a diabetic must pay close attention to how he feels and this transfer can be made if he listens to what his body tells him.

Many people have gotten completely off insulin as well as Goldenseal. Some people are put on insulin who are not true diabetics, as we have seen from the iris of the eyes. This type responds very fast and can overcome the use of both insulin and Goldenseal very rapidly. However, they must also be very careful to listen to their own bodies as the transfer is made from insulin to Goldenseal, as well as when to stop using Goldenseal. Diabetic test for blood sugar should be used daily as often as needed to monitor sugar levels.

NATURAL TECHNIQUE

A mild food diet and restricted oil intake is essential, with more vegetables than fruits in the beginning, and more cooked vegetables than raw. Make sure that all starch vegetables are baked at 500 degrees to change starch to glucose.

Vitamins:

A good multi-vitamin and mineral: used daily on a continuing basis

Calcium gluconate: to help the nervous system

B-complex: in addition to what is in the multiple, in high doses

Potassium: additional supply of this to help the kidneys. Approx. 4 - 99 mg. tablets daily.

Zinc, Manganese, and Chromium, are deficient in Diabetics and should be used in addition to the daily multiple and mineral.

Herbs: (adult doses listed; child's dose 9-14 years - 1/2 dose, 2-8 years - 1/3 dose)

Goldenseal root: to act as insulin (check blood sugar levels to determine amounts)

Juniper Berries: also act like a natural insulin. Can be used with goldenseal root or separately. Goldenseal root, however, has the ability to stop internal bleeding and so becomes a great deterrent of sight problems or skin problems.

Goldenseal root powder can be put directly on an open diabetic skin sore that will not heal and it will heal within a short time.

Herbal Pumpkin Formula:

Black Walnut - 1 part

Pumpkin Seed- 1 part

Sorrel- 1 part

Barefoot Root- 2 part

Tansy- 2 part

Bayberry- 2 part

(used not only to kill parasites but to keep the bowel clear. Most diabetic conditions have a chronic bowel condition, as is evident on the iris of the eyes.)
Approx. 6-8 capsules daily, 3-4 morning and 3-4 at night.

Psyllium: approx. 1 Tbs. twice daily may be used along with the Herbal Pumpkin formula.

Mothers do not realize the damage they do to their children when they allow them to consume so much sugar. Treats of this sort are not love, but rather unconcern or indulgence.

CHAPTER 8

ESSENTIAL KNOWLEDGE FOR PARENTS
VITAMINS, MINERALS, AND HERBS

How many times has your family felt sick in some way and rushed off to the doctor? He then suggests a list of drugs for you to take. By the time the doctor and pharmacists are through, the strain on your pocket book has made you even more ill. The drugs fail to do their job, make you drowsy, and often cause other side effects to your system. You are left to wonder if there isn't another way?

There is another way: In so many instances you can heal yourself with the proper selection of vitamins and minerals!

With this chapter, you can learn the daily doses of vitamins and minerals needed to improve your health; foods that can destroy certain vitamins; nutrients that will augment each vitamin; and the food and herbal sources for each vitamin. Name your illness or condition and you will find a vitamin or herbs that will improve your health.

When you finish this chapter, you will be excited about vitamins and minerals and you will be confident in feeling you now know how to use them.

A "vitamin from natural sources" generally means a concentrated food rich in a particular vitamin – with fat, moisture and fibers removed. Other factors in the concentrate the biochemists call "impurities", such things as the unknowns, the trace minerals, amino acids, enzymes, etc.

Occasionally the FDA will insist that certain known factors be excluded from supplements just because they are unproven. Because of the unresolved scientific dispute some known factors are excluded on these grounds alone. These known and unknown factors remain and exist in a more natural concentrate. If some of these factors are non-essential to you as they occur in nature, which is doubtful, you have nothing to lose. However, if they are essential, even though their function is yet unknown, it could possibly be critical to you.

The word natural has been used and abused until, like the word organic, much confusion exists as to the correct usage of the word. A definition of "natural" in its use here would be as they occur in nature naturally with both known and unknown factors existing, while a "synthetic" is created in the laboratory from so-called organic or inorganic substances unrelated to the foods in which the vitamins being produced would naturally occur. (A crystalline starts out as a natural and goes through a series of solvents until only the pure, isolated vitamin with none of the so-called impurities remain in crystalline form.)

The word organic has been much abused also from what the original organic gardener intended. Anything containing the carbon molecule today is considered organic, even coal or petroleum. The fact, however, that the words "natural" and "organic" have been much used and abused still leads everyone to believe that such things are becoming more and more important. It may even suggest that the scientists who have said there is no difference between organic and inorganic, synthetic or natural, are losing ground. What really counts in the long run is how such organic or inorganic, synthetic or natural, feels in the human body.

Cake, cigarettes, alcohol, coffee and candy didn't get the reputation for being unhealthy merely because someone said so. If a person says he does not smoke or drink, the other person will usually say, "Oh, you don't have any bad habits." Who told them they were bad habits? Why don't mothers and fathers give their babies coffee to drink for breakfast? Why do we keep a limit on the age to smoke and drink? How do people know these things are bad? Because of how it feels in the human body. We don't need any scientist to tell us so. If this is true, then it naturally follows that how the vitamins feel in the body is what counts, not what a scientist supposes it should do.

On a recent talk show a medical doctor called in to challenge me. He stated that more scientific research and blind studies needed to be done on herbs. My answer to him was that through the drug use and abuse period of the past 50 years or so, there had always been the counter culture of people who used herbs, vitamins and natural food. They have known how to combat and prevent disease and have known how it feels in the body to obey nature's rules, and somehow they didn't feel it was necessary to prove it to the world, even though they had proven it to themselves. He continued to challenge me, so my argument was: so what if science finds out what poisons me in a drug? How many ways can it hurt me for the few things it does? It does not seem logical to me to use such a dangerous substance, when I know how well I can feel with natural elements.

People who use natural vitamins and get results are not intimidated by illogical scientific argument. The people who have been really sick and have run the gauntlet of the drug method and somehow found their way to natural foods, natural vitamins and herbs, are the ones who do most proselyting for a healthier way because they have been there. They know first-hand the difference in how their bodies feel with one method or the other.

American citizens of today can boast 100 million cases of chronic disabling diseases. This is nearly half of the populations, and the other half works to support them. One in every 16 American aches with arthritis and rheumatism, not to mention the 250,000 children afflicted with arthritis. Every year more than a million people die of vascular disease. 97% of Americans have some kind of chronic dental disease. Who are we kidding with longevity statistics? There is a lot to be said for living while you are alive, and not living most of your life half dead.

Statistics lull us away into a false security because we are a rich nation, both in food and materials. We can afford to be charitable now, but what about hard times or famine with insufficient resources to maintain the institutions which house such people and pay welfare and disability payments? Could these statistics change under these circumstances? If American righteousness has kept up with its wealth, perhaps we could still be a charitable people. History does not convince us, however, that righteousness and wealth walk hand in hand. We are a sick nation. Autopsies performed on soldiers during the Korean war, with the average age of 22 years, revealed some degree of arteriosclerosis in over three-fourths of the cases. In 12% of these, arterial obstruction exceeded the 50% level – and this group was considered the best young people we had.

When America has the highest rate of infection per capita of any society, even higher than India, with all our sanitation practices, antibiotics and so-called "pharmaceutical advances", we need to take a long, hard look at how we feel; not what science keeps trying to persuade us to believe.

Many years ago my uncle, who was a horticulturist, ran his own private test when the new chemical fertilizers first came on the market. Taking two tomato plants and planting them side by side, with one stake between them on which they could both climb, having prepared the soil on the one side with chemical fertilizer and the other with organic matter compost, he began his vigil to see just what would happen. The plants began to grow, climbing the stake together, intertwining with one another. As they grew larger, he began to observe the difference in vigor beauty and health of the organically composted plant. He notices aphids beginning to come onto the plant feeding on the chemical ground. Strange how it didn't affect the stronger organic plant – what could he do to save the sick plant? The only thing he could have done – and this is the answer people find todayBspray it with poison to kill the bugs. Does this tell you anything?

The chemical companies have gradually become an enormous business. The arguments have vacillated between organic people and the chemical companies. The one thing that chemical growers could never argue with was taste and flavor – organic tastes better. Organic people claimed that people living on organic food were healthier because the food they were eating was healthier. The chemical farmer claimed that they could also grow food as large or larger and just as beautiful as anything grown with compost. Their biggest and best argument is, "Who could feed the world population on organically composted foods? It is too time consuming so leave us alone. We are at least getting the job done, providing for the world's peoples."

There has now developed a bridge between these two factions – a compromise that will eventually bless the world's people. Let me begin at the beginning. The balance of minerals has been so upset that it borders on insanity. It has gone so far it would take years to repair the situation, even with organic composting methods. Society cannot wait that long. Foods grown from depleted soil cannot be expected to be mineral rich.

We have made great strides in biological science that can presumably identify genes which cause learning disabilities. We have had so many brain-damaged and birth-defected children that our institutions are full to capacity. We spend an enormous amount of money each year to try to rehabilitate such children. Now the cry is that we need to stop producing such children. Thus, a mother can easily have a child aborted if she feels she cannot cope with such a disability.

We have coined two new words – brain dysfunction for the slow learning child and hyperactive or hyperkinetic for the too-busy-to-learn child. School systems, science and parents have decided that the way to control the learning for these types of children is to drug them. They are given speed or downers, like the illicit drugs found on the streets. Everyone seems to be concerned with the learning disability or acceptable behavior, but when a child is a nuisance or a menace, no one seems to be concerned with the child's silent agony. There have been no proofs as to the child's improved ability to learn by these methods. All that has been accomplished is to calm the hyperactive child so that the teacher and parent can stand them or salve the conscience of those who deal with the brain-dysfunctioned, into believing they are doing something for these behavioral misfits. The so-called technology to put a child in such a slot is so weak in its diagnosis and treatment, its masked secrecy only tends to enhance the mystical powers ascribed to the tester.

When will we learn to feed our children the necessary vitamins and minerals through good, live, whole foods from rich soil to solve these problems? America's sugar consumption is up to almost 150 lbs. per person per year. It was said several years ago that by 1980 one in five would be diabetic. The world, especially America, is drunk with sugar, not to mention all the other junk food. Our future generations will pay the price of our folly. We give our children baskets full of sugar for Easter, treats for Halloween, birthday cakes, candy for Christmas. Sugar is in almost every food that is put on the table.

The latest thing in agriculture today may be the saving factor: vegetation from the sea for mineral supplements and sea water for the plants instead of chemical fertilizers. Since all the ground has been so depleted that many of those who have argued that they can produce just as good a food as organic gardeners are realizing, that they have been mistaken. They have done a similar thing as the drug people have done.

Drugs do something in the body, it is certain; but they often work like whipping a tired horse, as with cortisone, until the gland is burned out, or they leave a residue that later becomes chronic disease like the tomato plant full of germs and parasites. The reason for this is because man was never intended to live on a mono-diet. All the foods that grow are widely spread with the minerals and vitamins he requires. He was never intended to eat the dirt or the rock, which is definition for "inorganic." Yet he fills his body with drugs made from potash rock and petroleum – inorganic by such standards, made from coal and salts from rock. When he uses all of these inorganic substances he is still much different from the plant who eats dirt or rock to grow, and doesn't care if it is chemical. If all the plant substances were broken down, as in compost, to become usable fuel for the plant, this would be nature's way and the best way.

The chemical fertilizer growers could have grown almost as well as the organic farmer if he had put in all the minerals. Since there are many unknowns in the vitamin business, how could he accomplish this? He made the big mistake of putting only three major chemicals in the ground.

These three are phosphorus, nitrates and potash. Potash may have contained some unknowns and extras, but most plants require 44 known minerals to be healthy. Some can get by with 35. Lettuce growers know they need an alkaline soil, and zinnia growers know it must be acidic.

The complex structures of plants must build on these 35 to 44 minerals to produce their own vitamins. When this cannot be achieved, the plant becomes diseased. What the chemical fertilizer people did not realize, was that by stimulating the growth with the major minerals they used, the plan would have to leach the soil to match the amounts so as to cause this greater growth demand created. This results in an eventual deficiency in the soil. When the soil has no natural replacements to build it up, this creates disease, the need for poison spray and also tasteless foods are created. What happens to people who live on such depleted food?

Now the bridge has been found between the organic gardener and the chemical fertilizer companies. Most companies are looking into the possibility of replacing the nutrients with sea water. This may save us for a while, but there is still the need for whole vegetation replacement back into the soil. In the meantime, wiser people realize the need for a good food supplement. This must be achieved in the only real place left on earth to find such essential nutrients – the sea and nature's wild untouched, uncultivated places. These healthful vitamins and minerals must be made with a base of sea vegetation and nature's wild uncultivated herbs.

VITAMINS

The minimum daily requirements, MDA, was used as a standard of the very smallest daily requirements to prevent deficiency. United States Recommended Daily Allowances, or RDA, means a standard set by the Food and Drug Administration. This standard has never been established as the complete fulfillment of nutritional requirements. Many nutrients have not been officially established. IU means international units and is used as a measure for Vitamins A, D, & E.

VITAMIN A (Antioxidant) (adult doses listed; child's dose 9-14 years - 1/2 dose, 2-8 years - 1/3 dose)
Daily dose - RDA - 5,000 IU
Approx. restore - 10,000 - 25,000 IU
Toxicity - 50,000 IU
Best source - Beta Carotene

Destroyed by:
alcohol
coffee
cortisone
excessive iron
mineral oil
Vitamin D deficiency

Part of the Body Essential For:

Eyes	hair
bones	soft tissue
teeth	lungs
synthesis of progesterone	utilization of protein

Symptoms of Deficiency:

night blindness	impaired vision
glued eyelids	dandruff
skin troubles	brittle nails & hair
acne, boils, impetigo	loss of hearing
loss of taste & smell	stone formations

psoriasis
warts
wrinkles
bone or joint pain
itchy, burning eyes
dry mouth
unable to store fat
Vitamin A poisoning
fatigue
abscesses in the ears
sinusitis
pink eye

gallstones
liver problems
red eyelids
corneal lesions
softening of the corneas
dry genitourinary system
hair loss
dry lips
insomnia
reproductive difficulties
frequent colds
pneumonia

Nutrients which Augment:
B Complex
Choline
Vitamins C, D, E
Calcium
Phosphorus
Zinc

Foods & Sources:
small amounts in all foods
1 peach 1,330 IU
watermelon
raw carrot juice
yellow & green foods
alfalfa
dandelion
okra pods
paprika
chickweed
gotu kola leaf
horseradish root
spirulina algae
cabbage
2 cantaloupe 9,240 IU

carrot - 1 med raw 10,000 IU
apricots - 3 dried 3,000 IU
kale
violets
red raspberries
grape leaves
cayenne
yellow dock
uva ursi leaf
peppermint leaf
senna leaf
beta carotene
spinach

a sprig of parsley contains as much vitamin A as a glass of carrot juice

Useful For:

body tissues repaired & maintained	gastrointestinal ulcers
	endometriosis
resists infection	preventing blindness
night vision	immune system
feeds the retina	slowing the aging process
Chronic Fatigue Syndrome	Guinne Barré
	Candida

The liver stores excess of Vitamin A, allowing it to be released as needed. Some conditions of the body such as liver disease and infection prohibit absorption of Vitamin A.

Toxic in large amounts (fish liver oil) – Beta Carotene not toxic in large amounts.

Mineral oil, when taken internally, carries away Vitamin A so it cannot be absorbed.

Higher doses are required during pregnancy & lactation – 6,000 - 8,000 IU.

Malnourishment or serious trauma are good reasons for high restoration doses of Vitamin A.

Vitamin A fights infection, and protects against colds and viruses. It is an antioxidant that helps protect the cells against cancer and other diseases by neutralizing free radicals.

VITAMIN B COMPLEX (Water soluble)
Daily dose - RDA - See individual B Vitamins
Approx. restore - See individual B Vitamins

Destroyed By:

birth control pills
coffee
stress
sugar

sulpha drugs
sleeping pills
infections
alcohol

Part of the Body Essential For:
eyes
gastrointestinal tract
hair
liver
mouth
ears
metabolism of
    carbohydrates,
    fat & protein

muscle tone
energy
blood
muscles
brain
soft tissue

Symptoms of Deficiency:
acne
anemia
constipation
high cholesterol
digestive problems
fatigue
hair (dull, falling out, dry)
dry skin
rough skin
insomnia
Alzheimer's

Nutrients which Augment:
Vitamin C
Calcium
Vitamin E
Phosphorus

Foods & Sources:
barley
bananas

figs
strawberries

watermelon
rutabagas
brussels sprouts
carrots
cauliflower
lettuce
cabbage
celery
cucumbers
lentils
leeks
mushrooms
almonds
brazil nuts
coconut
honey
molasses
alfalfa
artichokes
beans
 soy beans
broccoli
okra

parsley
avocados
cantaloupe
peaches
yogurt
potatoes
tomatoes
turnips
dates
oranges
corn
apples
raisins
peanuts
parsnips
peas
peppers
sauerkraut
wheat
rye
corn

Useful For:

alcoholism
allergies
baldness
heart abnormalities
hyperglycemia
migraine headaches
menstrual difficulties
hyperactive children
Chronic Fatigue syndrome
Epstein-Barr
Candida

psychosis
anemia
barbiturate overdose
cystitis
stress
overweight
Alzheimer's
Guinne Barré
Endometriosis
Parkinson's Disease

VITAMIN B1 (Thiamine) (Water soluble) (adult doses listed; child's dose 9-14 years - 1/2 dose, 2-8 years - 1/3 dose)
Daily dose B RDA B 50 mg.
Approx. restore - approx. 100 mg. daily

Destroyed By:
alcohol
sugar
clams
fever
birth control pills
sulfa drugs
coffee
stress
tobacco
antibiotics

Part of the Body Essential For:
brain
ears
eyes
hair
heart
nervous system
digestive tract
intestines
mental ability
to change glucose into energy or fat
memory vitamin
starch-sugar metabolism vitamin
resistance to noise & pain
production of hydrochloric acid

Symptoms of Deficiency:

anemia	nausea
sciatica	constipation
lumbago	slight paralysis
neuralgia	feet & hands numb

lack of hydrochloric acid
low blood pressure
low metabolic rate
poor coordination
edema
enlarged liver
tingling sensations
severe weight loss
general weakness
fatigue
loss of appetite
nervousness
labored breathing
asthma

irritability
forgetfulness
constipation
lactic acid build-up
pain, neuritis in legs
water-clogged heart
poor concentration
muscle atrophy
pain in knees
delayed ligament reflexes
beri-beri
starved thyroid
poor circulation

Nutrients Which Augment:
Vitamin B2
Folic Acid
B Complex
Niacin
Vitamins C, E
Manganese
Sulphur

Foods & Sources:
bladderwrack
dulse
kelp
fenugreek
grape leaves
red raspberries
okra
wheat germ
peas - 1 C = 4.5 mg
sunflower seeds - 1 C = 2.84 mg

whole wheat
asparagus
brown rice
potatoes
beans
green leafy vegetables
broccoli
most nuts
plums

Useful For:
alcoholism
congestive heart failure
anemia
nausea
mental illness
rapid heartbeat
stress
converting blood sugar to energy
new cell formation
muscles
increases oxygen to brain

Nervous tissue depends on Vitamin B1 for growth and development. Too much white flour and white rice can be the cause of a Thiamin deficiency. Every 100 grams of brown rice contains 2.93 mg. White rice for the same amount has only .60 mg.

Cooking vegetables in too much water, then throwing away the water causes a loss of Thiamin.

More is needed in older ages. Alcoholics can become very deficient. Brain damage can occur from a deficiency.

VITAMIN B2 Antioxidant (Riboflavin) (water soluble)
(adult doses listed; child's dose 9-14 years - 1/2 dose, 2-8 years - 1/3 dose)
Daily dose - RDA - 50 mg.
Approx. restore - 50-100 mg.

Destroyed By:
alcohol
sugar
clams
fever
ultraviolet rays
cooking
antibiotics

tranquilizers
oral contraceptives
light
tobacco
coffee
stress
strenuous exercise

Parts of the Body Essential For:
blood
nerves
bring oxygen to eyes
milk sugar or lactose increases
need for B2 unless fat is adequate in diet
cell respiration
metabolism of fats, carbohydrates and protein

Symptoms of Deficiency:
cracks at corner of mouth
whistle lines
loss of upper lip
swollen eyelids
sensitive to light
eyelids itch & burn
watery eyes
cataracts
insomnia
blood vessels close to skin, red as in alcoholism
glaucoma
bed sores
dizziness
poor night vision
bloodshot eyes
dermatitis
anemia
nervousness
poor digestion
liver impairment

hair loss

Nutrients Which Augment:
A
B Complex
B6
Niacin
Phosphorus
Vitamin C
Iron

Foods & Sources:

bladderwrack
dulse
fenugreek
kelp
saffron
wild rose hips
asparagus
beets
Brussel sprouts
broccoli
strawberries
avocados

lettuce
barley
asparagus root
nuts
watermelon
whole grains
peas
lima beans
sunflower seeds
carrots
cauliflower

Useful For:
acne
cataracts
mouth sores
itchy eyes
digestion
eye fatigue
dandruff
carpal tunnel syndrome

Riboflavin is essential for protein metabolism. A lack of B2 is one of the causes of birth defects such as skeletal abnormalities, abnormal development of bones such a cleft palate and jaw. It also causes pregnancy deficiencies.

The fetal damage potential is greater when certain drugs are taken. Even when the mother apparently has enough for herself, deficiency with the fetus can cause deformities.

VITAMIN B6 (Pyridoxine) (Water soluble)
(adult doses listed; child's dose 9-14 years - 1/2 dose, 2-8 years - 1/3 dose)
Daily dose - RDA - 50 mg.
Approx. restore - 50-100 mg.

Destroyed By:
birth control pills
coffee
alcohol
radiation
tobacco
freezing
storage
canning
processing grains
cooking

Parts of the Body Essential For:
Essential to use fatty acids, linoleic acids & amino acids from
    protein
assists in hormonal metabolism of thyroid, pancreas & adrenal
    glands
antibody formation
digestion
fat & protein utilization
maintains sodium & potassium balance
necessary for synthesis of DNA & RNA
necessary for production of hydrochloric acid
needed for normal brain function
promotes red blood cell formation

Symptom of Deficiency:
eczema in babies
acne, psoriasis
skin dermatitis
wrinkles
sore mouth
fainting easily
muscle cramps
bed wetting
bladder retention
tooth decay
sinus problem
water retention
toxemia in pregnancy
Guinne Barré
anemia
convulsions
headache
flaky skin
sore tongue
rheumatism
depression
fatigue
weak memory
hair loss
hearing problems
B6 levels decline with age
numbness
nausea in pregnancy - up to 250 mg.
motion sickness - up to 250 mg.
irradiation sickness - up to 250 mg.
arthritis
tingling sensations
hemorrhoids
ear noise
sea sickness
colitis
vomiting

anorexia

Nutrients Which Augment:
B Complex
B1
B2
Pantothenic Acid
Vitamin C
Magnesium
Potassium
Sodium

Foods & Sources:

asparagus
beets
Brussel sprouts
carrots
cauliflower
lettuce
barley
bananas
whole grains
walnuts
filberts
watermelon
dulse
all foods contain some

peas
cabbage
corn
potatoes
figs
fish
bananas
avocados
spinach
peanuts
sunflower seeds
wheat germ
strawberries

Useful For:
prevention of arteriosclerosis
baldness
mental retardation
muscular disorders
nervousness
stress
overweight
sensitivity to light or sun
skin problems

cancer immunity
cholesterol
diuretic
PMS
allergies
arthritis
asthma
anorexia
kidney stones
carpal tunnel syndrome

More Vitamin B6 is needed during pregnancy and old age. Leg cramps during pregnancy are thought to be a lack in calcium and magnesium. Often it is the lack of B6.

VITAMIN B12 (Cyanocobalamin-Cobalt) (Water soluble)
(adult doses listed; child's dose 9-14 years - 1/2 dose, 2-8 years - 1/3 dose)
Daily dose - RDA - 50 mcg.
Approx. restore - 50-100 mcg.

Destroyed By:
alcohol
coffee
laxatives
tobacco

Parts of the Body Essential For:
glands
phenobarbital & dilantin & heat destroy folic acid. Folic acid is
    necessary to use B12. This is a good reason for using raw
    cold-pressed oils & raw fruits and nuts
essential in use of meat protein
to prevent anemia
essential to gland restoration where meat is used
blood
nerves
Symptoms of Deficiency:

abdominal difficulties
nausea
gas
diarrhea
fatigue
constipation
hallucinations
sleepiness
headaches
pernicious anemia
nervousness
moodiness
labored breathing
menstrual disturbances
back stiffness & pain
painful & burning eyelids
vaginal itching
loss of distance vision
red scaly spots between nose & lips
pale, white lips
poor appetite
ringing in ears
spots before eyes
enlarged liver & spleen
chronic fatigue
Epstein-Barr
depression
enlargement of liver
digestive disorders
dizziness
vomiting
pain
drowsiness
memory loss
inability to produce hydrochloric acid
heart failure
sore mouth
 swollen tongue

bright red, painful tongue
spinal cord degeneration
irritability

Nutrients Which Augment:
B Complex
B6
Choline
Inositol
Vitamin C
Potassium
Sodium
Folic Acid
Iron

Foods & Sources:
sea vegetation
dulse
kelp
soy products

Useful For:
alcoholism
allergies
arthritis
bronchial asthma
irregular menstrual periods
stress
bursitis
epilepsy

BIOTIN (Vitamin H) (Water soluble - part of B Complex)
Daily dose - RDA - 150-300 mcg.
Approx. restore - 300-500 mcg.
(adult doses listed; child's dose 9-14 years - 1/2 dose, 2-8 years - 1/3 dose)

Destroyed By:

alcohol
coffee
raw egg white
antibiotics
sulpha drugs
saccharin

Parts of the Body Essential For:
hair
cell growth
cell longevity
vitamin B utilization
metabolism of carbohydrates, fats, and proteins
fatty acid production

Symptoms of Deficiency:
dry skin
gray skin
muscular pain
loss of appetite
eczema
dermatitis
high blood sugar
insomnia
sore tongue
leg cramps
mental depression
heart pain
hands & feet tingle
pallor
anemia
depression

Nutrients Which Augment:
B Complex
B12
Folic Acid
Vitamin C

Sulphur

Foods & Sources:
soy beans, 1 C = 120 mcg
lentils, 1 C = 25 mcg
bean sprouts, 1 C = 200 mcg
brown rice
rolled oats
nuts

Useful For:
baldness
dermatitis
eczema
leg cramps
healthy hair and skin
cradle cap in infants
relieves muscle pain
promotes healthy sweat glands
promotes healthy nerve tissue
promotes healthy bone marrow

CHOLINE (Part of B Complex) (Water soluble)
Daily dose - RDA - None
Approx. restore - 1,000-10,000 mcg
(adult doses listed; child's dose 9-14 years - 1/2 dose, 2-8 years - 1/3 dose)

Destroyed By:
sugar (excessive)
coffee
alcohol
anti-histamines
anti-depressants
Parts of the Body Essential For:
keeps arteries clear
lecithin formation
liver, gall bladder regulation

metabolism (fats & cholesterol)
nerve transmission
thymus

Symptoms of Deficiency:
Without choline, cholesterol reaches high levels because it takes choline to produce lecithin. Damage to kidneys result from lack of choline when protein diet is used.

Nutrients Which Augment:
Vitamins A, B Complex, B12
Folic Acid
Linoleic Acid
Inositol
Lecithin

Foods & Sources:
soy oil
wheat germ oil
lecithin
soybeans
whole grain cereals

Useful For:
alcoholism
arteriosclerosis
baldness
high cholesterol
constipation
dizziness
ear noise
diseases of the nervous system
Parkinson's disease
Huntington's disease
viral hepatitis
high blood pressure
hardening of the arteries
heart trouble

headaches
kidney impairment
gastric ulcers
manic depression
liver impairment
stunted growth
memory loss
hepatitis
hypoglycemia
insomnia
inability to digest fats

Mother's milk has a choline-lecithin balance for humans, which cows milk does not. Therefore, nursing mothers give their children an immune ability which a bottle fed baby does not have.

Choline has an effect on the thymus glands also, which in turn has something to do with growth and immune response in a child. Elevates the HDL Cholesterol (Good cholesterol) level.

FOLIC ACID (Part of B Complex) (Water soluble)
Daily dose - RDA - 400 mcg
Approx. restore - 1,000-10,000 mcg
(adult doses listed; child's dose 9-14 years - 1/2 dose, 2-8 years - 1/3 dose)

Destroyed By:
birth control pills
alcohol
coffee
stress
tobacco
cooking, dissolves in water
air
light
cooking

Parts of the Body Essential For:

synthesis of DNA & other nucleic acids
appetite
body growth & reproduction
protein metabolism, red blood cell formation
growth of cells
strengthening immune system
energy production
brain food

Symptoms of Deficiency:
anemia
digestive disturbances
graying hair
growth problems
pregnancy cap
skin dryness
joints dry
diarrhea
afterbirth hemorrhage
mental illness and/or paranoia
depression anxiety
sore - red tongue
birth defects
weakness
apathy
fatigue
insomnia
labored breathing
memory problems

Nutrients Which Augment:
B Complex
B12
Biotin
Pantothenic Acid
Vitamin C

Foods & Sources:

dates, 1 med = 2500 mcg
spinach, 1 C = 448 mcg
wheat bran
beet greens
kale
endive
barley
asparagus
turnips
potatoes
broccoli
black-eyed peas
lima beans
green leafy vegetables
orange juice
swiss chard

Useful For:
alcoholism
diarrhea
fatigue
mental illness
stomach ulcers
stress
baldness
anemia
arteriosclerosis
healing
Elderly people suffer from deficiency.
angina (pain in heart)

400mcg. before conception and after pregnancy - (vital for normal fetal development and premature birth.)

Deficiency may be linked to inadequate consumption of fresh fruits and vegetables since cooking destroys this vitamin.

INOSITOL (Part of B Complex) (Water Soluble)

Daily dose - RDA -- none

Approx. restore - 100-1,000 mg

(adult doses listed; child's dose 9-14 years - 1/2 dose, 2-8 years - 1/3 dose)

Destroyed By:
alcohol
coffee
caffeine

Parts of the Body Essential For:
lecithin formation
metabolism of fats
hair growth
reduces cholesterol
retards artery hardening
has an inhibiting factor in cancer
has been used for nerve damage in MS, but must be used in
    conjunction with Vitamin E
when used with choline, breaks up fat
removes fat from the liver

Symptoms of Deficiency:
high cholesterol
eczema
hair loss
eye problems
constipation
irritability
mood swings
skin exceptions

Nutrients Which Augment:
B Complex
B12
Choline
Linoleic acid
Vitamin E

Foods & Sources:
wheat germ
oranges, 1 med = 400 mg
grapefruit, 1 med = 500 mg
brown rice
citrus fruit
molasses
fruits
vegetables
whole grains

Useful For:
arteriosclerosis
baldness
high cholesterol
heart disease
overweight
calming
anxiety
insomnia

NIACIN (Vitamin B3, Part of B Complex) (Water soluble)
Daily Dose - RDA - 50 mg
Approx. restore - 50-100 mg
(adult doses listed; child's dose 9-14 years - 1/2 dose, 2-8 years - 1/3 dose)

Destroyed By:
alcohol
antibiotics
coffee
corn sugar
excessive starch
cooking

Parts of the Body Essential For:
circulation

reduces cholesterol
growth
hydrochloric acid production
metabolism of proteins, carbohydrates, & starches
sex hormone production
healthy skin
synthesis of sex hormones
normal secretion of bile and stomach fluids

Symptoms of Deficiency:
appetite loss
canker sores
depression
insomnia
muscle weakness
nausea
skin eruptions
nervous problems
inflamation
coated tongue
impaired memory
schizophrenia
dementia
fear
neuralgia
diarrhea
tongue deep red with fissures, (fissures will turn black if great
    deficiency)becomes pellagra or Black Tongue (plague)
indigestion
fatigue
halitosis
rash on neck & forearms
dizziness
Alzheimer's
low blood sugar
headaches
limb pains

Nutrient Which Augment:
B Complex
Vitamins B1, B2, C
Phosphorus

Foods & Sources:
whole wheat
sunflower seeds, 1 C = 7.8 mg
peas, 1 C = 3.7 mg

Useful For:
senility
cataracts
acne
baldness
halitosis
high blood pressure
leg cramps
migraine headache
tooth decay
memory enhancer

Niacin dilates blood vessels and causes hot flashes. It is used to increase circulations to the brain in senility, schizophrenia and ear and eye problems. Flush free niacin is not as effective - flush or Hot flash is needed to bring oxygen to the brain.

It is also useful for alcoholics and reduces cholesterol levels. It has been used to treat pellagra, black tongue and fissure of the tongue. Women are more subject to this than men.

PANTOTHENIC ACID Antioxidant
(Part of B Complex - anti-stress vitamin) (Water soluble)
Daily Dose - RDA - .05 - 10 mg
Approx. restore - 50-100 mg
(adult doses listed; child's dose 9-14 years - 1/2 dose, 2-8 years - 1/3 dose)

Destroyed By:
coffee
alcohol
methyl bromide

Parts of the Body Essential For:
anti-body formations
carbohydrate, fat & protein conversion to energy
vitamin utilization
lymph glands
adrenal
tonsils
metabolism

Symptoms of Deficiency:
arthritis
nausea
tingling in the hands
cataracts
low blood pressure
swollen glands
glaucoma
gastritis
ulcers
gout
muscle cramps
stretch marks
anxiety
fatigue
hypoglycemia
exhaustion
blackouts
headaches
nervousness
dizziness
digestive problems
depression
colitis

grinding teeth

Nutrients Which Augment:
B Complex
Vitamins B6, B12, C
Biotin
Folic Acid
PABA

Foods & Sources:
whole wheat & bran
elderberries, 1 C = 82 mg
orange juice, 1 C = 45 mg
sesame seeds
althea root
soy beans
peas
brewers yeast
sunflower seeds
capsicum
all bright
red raspberry leaf
spirulina algae
asparagus
cabbage
fever few leaf
ginkgo biloba leaf
hops

Useful For:
allergies
baldness
detoxifying alcohol in the bloodstream
gray hair
reducing negative effects of aging
used as a fumigator
important during high stress periods acts as a stamina enhancer
protection against cardiovascular disease

cystitis
digestive disorders
stress
tooth decay
hypoglycemia
relief of gas
arthritis
promotes healing
cold sores
sinus
asthma
respiratory flu
colds

PABA (Para-Amino-Benzoic-Acid B Part of B Complex) (Water soluble)
Daily Dose - RDA - 50
Approx. restore - 50-100 mg
(adult doses listed; child's dose 9-14 years - 1/2 dose,
2-8 years - 1/3 dose)

Destroyed by:
alcohol
coffee
sulfa drugs

Parts of the Body Essential For:
blood cell formation
gray hair restoration
headaches
irritability
maintenance of healthier intestinal flora breakdown and
    utilization of proteins

Symptoms of Deficiency:
digestive disturbances
graying hair
irritability

fatigue
depression
nervousness
patchy areas
white skin
fatigue

Nutrients Which Augment:
B Complex
Folic acid
Vitamin C
Pantothenic acid

Foods & Sources:
black strap molasses
wheat germ
spinach
whole grains

PABA can only be synthesized by intestinal bacteria & stimulates intestinal bacteria to produce folic acid. It is also involved somehow in the utilization of Pantothenic acid.

Useful For:
baldness
gray hair
overactive thyroid
parasitic disease
fatigue
burns
dry skin
sunburn
wrinkles
skin spots
skin cancer
rheumatic fever
stress
infertility

Rocky Mtn. Spotted Fever, approx. 1,000 mg daily
hair color restored - approx 200 mg after each meal
PABA performs the same thing in the body that sulfa drug does, killing bacteria, without the side effects of sulfa: extreme fatigue, anemia, eczema

PANGAMIC ACID (Part of B Complex – B15 – not sold in US at present)
Daily Dose - RDA - none
Approx. restore - not known
(adult doses listed; child's dose 9-14 years - 1/2 dose, 2-8 years - 1/3 dose)

Destroyed by:
alcohol
coffee

Parts of the Body Essential For:
cell oxidation and respiration
metabolism of proteins, fats & starches
glandular & nervous system stimulation

Symptoms of Deficiency:
heart problems
nervousness
gland malfunction

Nutrients Which Augment:
B Complex
Vitamins C, E

Foods & Sources:
brown rice
seeds - sunflower, pumpkin, sesame
almonds

Useful For:
alcoholism

asthma
arteriosclerosis
high cholesterol
emphysema
heart disease
headache
insomnia
poor circulation
premature aging
shortness of breath
rheumatism

VITAMIN C Antioxidant (Ascorbic acid) (Water soluble)
Daily dose - RDA - 45 mg
Approx. restore - 250-5,000 mg
(adult doses listed; child's dose 9-14 years - 1/2 dose, 2-8 years - 1/3 dose)

Destroyed By:
antibiotics
aspirin
cortisone
stress
tobacco
alcohol
antidepressants
analgesics
anticoagulants
birth control pills
steroids

Parts of the Body Essential For:
bone and teeth formation
digestion
red blood cell formation
prevents hemorrhage
resists shock & colds
cell respiration

breaking down protein
healing
capillary
cartilage & connective tissue
adrenal gland function
aids in production of anti-stress hormones and interferon

Symptoms of Deficiency:
anemia
varicose veins
hepatitis, liver
cataracts
glaucoma
high blood pressure
ulcers
arthritis, gout
high cholesterol
rheumatic fever
weakness in arteries
low blood pressure
nosebleed
loose teeth
bleeding membranes (mouth, red toothbrush)
scurvy
bruise easily
lack of energy
cold sores
adrenal exhaustion
edema
mononucleosis
wounds will not heal
disc problems
joint pains
pigmentation during pregnancy
increased risk of colds & infections
poor digestion

Nutrients Which Augment:

All vitamins & minerals
Bioflavonoid
calcium
magnesium
Folic
increases absorption of iron
pycnogenol
grape seed extract

Foods & Sources:
oranges, 1 med = 100 mg
broccoli, 1 C = 135 mg
green peppers, 1 med = 100 mg
grapefruit, 1 med = 100 mg
papaya, raw, 225 mg
strawberries, 1 C = 90 mg
avocados
dulse
althea root
horseradish root
broccoli
cauliflower
lemons
rosehips fruit
papayas
all fruits & most vegetables

Useful For:
sore throat, strep
sinusitis
stress
aspirin poisoning
black widow spider bites
poison oak or ivy
carbon monoxide poisoning
radiation poisoning
broken bones
bruises

burns
poisonous bites
meningitis
encephalitis
virus diseases
swollen glands
polio
asthma
respiratory ailments
acute sinusitis
kidney infection
phlebitis
hay fever
colds
barrier against bladder cancer
enhances immune system
promotes healing of wounds and burns
reduces cholesterol
high blood pressure
atherosclerosis
protects against blood clotting
endometriosis
Chronic Fatigue Syndrome
Guinne Barré
cancer
Epstein-Barr

There are many arguments about how man is missing a gene that requires him to get all of his Vitamin C out of his food, since other mammals produce their own Vitamin C plentifully. If science would recognize that man lives better as a fruitarian he could suppose that was why he was made in such a way that would make Vitamin C production unnecessary in his body.

When a person can't digest there vitamins - taking extra vitamin C will help them digest and utilize their vitamins.

If man took the comparison amounts that other animals produce, he would have to take 20,000 mg. a day. The RDA is only 60 mg. Man was intended to be a fruit eater and if he were, he would probably not need so much Vitamin C to compensate for the stress foods he lives on.

It has been agreed upon by experts that stress destroys Vitamin C and that under stress the adrenal glands output of hormones increases. Collagen or connective tissue requires Vitamin C. Man's body cannot make collagen without Vitamin C. This is why additional Vitamin C is so helpful to the healing process from surgery or injury when tissue repair is essential.

Vitamin C's main function is the reason it detoxifies even the worst poisons – because it dissolves mucus waste and carries it off through the kidneys. Toxic poisons become a part of mucus waste and Vitamin C quickly detoxifies the body from an acid to an alkaline. This is proven in that a cold can be brought on by taking high doses of Vitamin C, breaking up and moving waste from the body. It also has an antibiotic ability to destroy germs.

When Vitamin C is taken in large doses for extended periods, such as a five to ten days, calcium and Vitamin B should be added, as the Vitamin C leaches these elements and caused nervousness and hollow, easily broken bones.

There has been much discussion about Vitamin C. It has been my experience, and the experience of many other that when Vitamin C is issued (1,000 mg. an hour) in acute illnesses such as a cold, etc., it dissolves mucus and usually stops acute disease or inflammation within a day or two. It has been used successfully even with small babies.

Vitamin C has been considered to be harmful to the kidney when taken in high doses. Certainly it is when it is a coal tar product. Taking high doses of coal tar would be very harmful. To determine whether or not your Vitamin C is a coal tar product, you can make this experiment: Place the tablet or powder on a teaspoon with water, hold over the burner of the stove and let it boil. If it boils away to a white powder, it is not a coal tar product. If it boils to a sticky, black gum, it is a coal tar product. Vitamin C has recently been made from wood, and of course, would be synthetic. When made from corn and citrus, it is a natural food product.

When used in the case of a cold or acute disease, it should be determined just how the Vitamin C you use is made, or you will not get the results. Could this be the reason for the controversy about Vitamin C? I have found where acute disease is present, straight ascorbic acid is best, usually taking it only a day or two, as it dissolves mucus rapidly. Any acute disease brings with it a rapid pulse, as waste is on the move in the blood. High doses of Vitamin C often increases the heartbeat, as with acute disease. The addition of approximately one capsule of cayenne will usually slow down and smooth out the heart. Bioflavonoid Vitamin C is best for a daily dose.

With twenty-five 500 milligram tablets, liquified with one-eighth cup warm water each teaspoon will equal 1,000 mg; add honey to taste.

Polio virus has been stopped in 72 hours with Vitamin C therapy. We have too long starved the diabetic of fruit sugars and accompanying Vitamin C which would stop the inflammation and running ulcers that seem to go with later stages of diabetes.

VITAMIN D (Sunshine vitamin) (Fat soluble)
Daily Dose - RDA - 400 IU
Approx. restore - 500-1,500 IU
(adult doses listed; child's dose 9-14 years - 1/2 dose, 2-8 years - 1/3 dose)

Destroyed By:
mineral oil
cortisone
antacids

Parts of the Body Essential For:

Calcium & phosphorous metabolism
bone formation
heart action
blood clotting
skin respiration
teeth
growth

People who do not get out in the sunshine do themselves a great injustice because sunshine is required to ensure adequate amounts of vitamin D in the body; much mental illness is caused from lack of calcium, and calcium cannot be utilized without Vitamin D

Symptoms of Deficiency:
burning mouth & throat
insomnia
myopia
nervousness
poor metabolism
soft bones & teeth
fingernail split & deep lines
rickets
high cholesterol
muscle cramps
loss of appetite
diarrhea
visual problems
weakness
enlarged joints
bowed legs
faulty jaw development
retarded growth
joint and back pain
bones break easily
osteoporosis
hypoglycemia
weight loss
pyorrhea

backache
acne

Nutrients Which Augment:
Vitamins A, C, F
Calcium
Phosphorus
Choline

Foods & Sources:
alfalfa
sunlight
lettuce

Useful for:
alcoholism
arthritis
stress
counteracts drug harm

Vitamin D is stored by the body in the liver during the winter months.

VITAMIN E Antioxidant (Tocopherol) (Fat soluble)
Daily Dose - RDA - 100 IU
Approx. restore - 100-600 IU
d-alpha tocopherol
(adult doses listed; child's dose 9-14 years - 1/2 dose,
2-8 years - 1/3 dose)

Destroyed By:
estrogen drugs
birth control pills
chlorine
mineral oil
rancid fats & oils
inorganic iron

Parts of the Body Essential For:
aging retardation
anti-clotting factor
lowers cholesterol
strengthens capillary walls
fertility
muscle, nerve maintenance
growth
nutrition
essential to use of Vitamins A, C, D, & K
protects fat tissue from abnormal breakdown as in diabetes
effective in menopause
effective in menstrual cramps
heart
normal blood pressure
effective on burns & scars
healing broken bones
increases oxygen
improves circulation

Symptoms of Deficiency:
sterility and infertility
blood clots
bowel and breast cancer
detachment of retina
heart problems
anemia
nervousness
miscarriage
puffy eyes
menopause problems
varicose veins
Parkinson's Disease

Caution: chronic heart (coronary artery disease) approx. 800 to 1,600 IU daily, rheumatic heart approx. 90 IU for 3-4 weeks. Then increase to 150 IU. High blood pressure requires careful supervision. Slow results in beginning with eventual great value.

Nutrients Which Augment:
Vitamins A, B1, B, C, F
Manganese
Phosphorus
Inositol
Selenium (trace element)
Zinc

Foods & Sources:
wheat germ oil, 1 T ' 40 IU
safflower oil, 1 T ' 20 IU
nettle leaves, 1 lb ' 98.2
oats
broccoli
rice
green leafy vegetables

Useful For:
detached retina
premature babies
anemia
hernia
muscle weakness
crossed eyes
miscarriages
burns & scars
varicose veins
frostbite
pain
congenital heart disease
acne
cancer cell growth
skin cancer
hemophilia
sinusitis
arthritis
colitis

arteriosclerosis
maintaining youth
hot flashes
drug abuse
leg cramps
Chronic Fatigue Syndrome
Guinne Barré
Epstein Barr
endometriosis
PMS
reduces high blood pressure
preventing cataracts
gallstones
hepatitis
clots
heart attack
thyroid gland
stomach ulcers
Candida
elimination of poisons
energy & endurance

VITAMIN F (Unsaturated fatty acid) (Fat soluble)
Daily Dose - none
Approx. restore - 10% total calorie intake
(adult doses listed; child's dose 9-14 years - 1/2 dose,
2-8 years - 1/3 dose)

Destroyed By:
radiation
X-ray

Parts of the Body Essential For:
prevents hardening of arteries
normalizes blood pressure
gland activity

Symptoms of Deficiency:

acne
brittle nails
eczema
gall stones
brittle hair
underweight
varicose veins

Nutrients Which Augment:
Vitamins A, C, D, E
Phosphorus

Foods & Sources:
vegetable oils
wheat germ
sunflower seeds

Useful For:
allergies
baldness
bronchial asthma
eczema
gallbladder problems
leg ulcers
psoriasis
overweight
rheumatoid arthritis

VITAMIN K (Menadione) (Fat soluble)
Daily dose -- RDA – 100mcg
Approx. restore B 300-500 mcg
(adult doses listed; child's dose 9-14 years - 2 dose,
2-8 years - 1/3 dose)

Destroyed By:
drugs
aspirin
antibiotics

mineral oils
radiation
rancid fats
X-rays

Parts of the Body Essential For:
clotting of blood
bone formation and repair

Symptoms of Deficiency:
hemophilia
hemorrhages easily
nosebleeds
diarrhea

Nutrients Which Augment:
are not known

Foods & Sources:

green leafy vegetables	cabbage
safflower oil	cauliflower
soy beans	plantain
alfalfa	tomatoes
chestnuts	peas
shepherds purse	spinach
carrots	potatoes

Useful for:
bruising
eye hemorrhage
gall stones
menstrual problems
preparing for childbirth
hemorrhage

Vitamin K is synthesized or manufactured by intestinal bacteria. It is, therefore necessary to maintain natural flora in the bowel - antibiotics destroy this flora.

Vitamin K is used when patient has been on long term antibiotics of intravenous feeding for more than seven days.

VITAMIN P (Bioflavonoids)
Daily Dose - RDA - none
Approx. restore - 300-3,000 mg
(adult doses listed; child's dose 9-14 years - 1/2 dose,
2-8 years - 1/3 dose)

Destroyed By:
antibiotics
aspirin
cortisone
stress
tobacco
alcohol
antidepressants
analgesics
anticoagulants
birth control pills steroids

Parts of the Body Essential For:
blood vessel walls
connective tissue
skin
prevention of flu & colds
strengthens capillaries
minimizes bruising

Symptoms of Deficiency:
same as Vitamin C
uterine bleeding
irregular menstrual flow where no other cause is known
varicose veins

Nutrients Which Augment:
Vitamin C

Foods & Sources:
buckwheat
apricots
tomatoes
cherries
green peppers
paprika
cantaloupe
broccoli
blue-green algae
papaya
black currants
skins & pulp of fruits: (white material just beneath the peel of citrus fruits)

Useful For:

pain relief

asthma

bleeding gums

colds

eczema

dizziness

high blood pressure

miscarriage

rheumatic fever

lower cholesterol

oral herpes

ulcers

hemorrhoids

veins

capillaries

bruises

antibacterial effect

rheumatism

RH babies to strengthen veins & arteries for blood change

The rest of the C-Complex necessary on a daily intake of minimum dose – used as a preventative. Straight Vitamin C (ascorbic acid) in high doses work faster for acute disease, but the full C-Complex should be used on a regular basis.

MINERALS

CALCIUM
Daily Dose - RDA - 800-1,400 mg
Approx. restore - 1,000-2,000 mg
Best Source - Gluconate or lactate
(adult doses listed; child's dose 9-14 years - 1/2 dose, 2-8 years - 1/3 dose)

Destroyed By:
lack of exercise
stress
antacids containing aluminum
alcohol
oxalate-rich Foods & Sources:
cooked spinach
rhubarb
green peppers

Parts of the Body Essential For:
bone & tooth formation
blood clotting
heart rhythm
healthy gums
nerve tranquilizing
nerve transmission
muscle growth & contraction
lactation & pregnancy
oxygen to brain
to maintain proper permeability of cell membrane

Symptoms of Deficiency:

menstrual cramps	pasty complexion
cyst formations	numbness arms & or legs
tooth decay	brooding, complaining
night sweats	nervousness
leg cramps	heart palpitations
mental depression	elevated blood cholesterol
irritability	hyperactivity
rheumatoid arthritis	aching joints

brittle nails
Alzheimer's
sores do not heal
lack of courage
soft bones
deterioration of spine
sleeplessness
muscle cramps

tooth decay
tooth grinding
eczema
rickets
insomnia
hypertension
Parkinson's Disease

Nutrients Which Augment:
Vitamins A, C, D, F
Iron
Magnesium
Manganese
Phosphorus
Boron
Lysine

Foods & Sources:
artichokes
lima beans
okra
rutabaga
sauerkraut
squash
whole wheat bread
hominy
figs
peaches
parsley
parsnips
peas
potatoes
rhubarb
tomatoes
turnips, tops & root
carob
beans

beets, leaves & root
broccoli
watercress
rye bread
corn
rice
rye
nettle leaf
bananas
sesame
walnuts
asparagus
cauliflower
endive
blueberries
buchu
tahini
wheat
apples

hickory nuts
raspberries
olives
oranges
avocados
cabbage
kelp
Brussel sprouts

raisins
dates
carrots
celery
bayberry bark
white oak bark
par d'arco bark

Useful For:

arthritis
backache
insomnia
pain
heart
kidney
muscles
menopause
cancer
bites
spleen
hair
rheumatism
lowering cholesterol levels
preventing cancer
immune system
preventing osteoporosis
Chronic Fatigue Syndrome

aging symptoms
foot & leg cramps
menstrual cramps
dental pain
skin
brain
liver
overweight
delivery
broken bones
bones
teeth
Guinne Barré
cardiovascular disease
lowering blood pressure
endometriosis
provides energy
Epstein-Barr

CHROMIUM

Daily Dose - RDA- none
Approx. restore - 100-300 mcg. Best source - Picolinate
(adult doses listed; child's dose 9-14 years - 1/2 dose, 2-8 years - 1/3 dose)

Destroyed By:
refined foods
strenuous exercise

Parts of the Body Essential For:
normal blood sugar levels
glucose metabolism

Symptoms of Deficiency:
arteriosclerosis
glucose intolerance in diabetes
growth inhibited
high cholesterol
hyperglycemia
hypoglycemia

Nutrients Which Augment:
Vitamin C

Foods & Sources:
sea vegetation
corn oil
grains
fresh fruits & vegetables
butchers broom root
catnip herb
damiana leaf
ginkgo biloba leaf
hibiscus flower
horsetail herb
hydrangea root
juniper berries
milk thistle leaf
nettle leaf
oat grass straw

passion flower
horseradish root
potatoes
red clover
senna leaf
thyme leaf
yarrow herbs
dulse
barley grass
buchu
lemon grass
burdock root
dried beans

Useful For:
diabetes
affects insulin drug requirement
improvement of insulin balance
lowers blood sugar levels
energy

coronary artery disease
osteoporosis
lowers cholesterol when used with Vitamin C
reduces body fat & helps to build lean muscle

COBALT (Trace mineral)
Daily Dose- RDA 100 mcg
Approx. restore - 100-300 mcg
(adult doses listed; child's dose 9-14 years - 1/2 dose,
2-8 years - 1/3 dose)

Destroyed By:
Not known

Parts of the Body Essential For:
Not known

Symptoms of Deficiency:
pernicious anemia
slow growth
anemia
nervous disorder

Nutrients Which Augment:
Vitamin B12
Folic acid

Foods & Sources:
wheat germ
comfrey leaves

Useful For:
pregnancy
lactation

COPPER (Trace mineral)
Daily Dose - RDA - 2 mg

Approx. restore - 2-4 mg
(adult doses listed; child's dose 9-14 years - 1/2 dose, 2-8 years - 1/3 dose)

Destroyed By:
zinc – high intake

Parts of the Body Essential For:
bone formation
hair & skin color
healing processes
hemoglobin & blood cell formation
energy production

Symptoms of Deficiency:
general weakness
impaired respiration
skin sores
gray hair
anemia
diarrhea
osteoporosis

Nutrients Which Augment:
Cobalt
Vitamin C
Iron
Zinc

Foods & Sources:

brazil nuts, 4 mg	filberts
soybeans, 1 C = 2 mg	widespread in all foods
almonds	kidney beans
prunes	apricots
lima beans	avocado
broccoli	corn
wheat bran	figs
currents	navy beans

Useful For:
anemia
baldness
formation of collagen

Copper accumulates in the blood when there is no iron, eventually causing Wilson's Disease

IODINE
Daily Dose - RDA - 100-130 mcg
Approx. restore - 100-1,000 mcg
Best source - dulse or kelp
(adult doses listed; child's dose 9-14 years - 1/2 dose, 2-8 years - 1/3 dose)

Destroyed By:
Vitamin C - take 8 hours apart

Parts of the Body Essential For:
hair
skin
teeth
nails
speech
mentality

Symptoms of Deficiency:
cold hands & feet
dry hair
irritability
nervousness
can lead to breast cancer
fatigue
obesity
difficult birth
hardening of arteries
goiter

Nutrients Which Augment:
Sodium – necessary for the use of iodine

Food & Sources:
sea vegetation
turnips, root
peppers
kelp
dulse-deep sea lettuce
carrots
raw goat milk
spinach
potatoes
beans
chard
broccoli
garlic
turnip greens
asparagus

Useful For:
arteriosclerosis
hair problems
goiter
hyperthyroidism
helps to metabolize excess fat
childbirth
lactation
infection
inflammation
destroying unfriendly bacteria in the body
Deficiency in pregnant mother can cause mongoloids or mental retardation in unborn child & cretinism
losses occur during summer - perspiration

IRON
Daily Dose - RDA -10-18 mg
Approx. restore - 15-50 mg

(adult doses listed; child's dose 9-14 years -1/2 dose, 2-8 years -
1/3 dose)

Destroyed By:
pain drugs
coffee
excess phosphorus
tea
zinc – excessive
strenuous exercise, heavy perspiration
prolonged use of antacids
long-term illness

Parts of the Body Essential For:
disease resistance
muscles
blood
hemoglobin
oxygen
bone marrow
healthy immune system

Symptoms of Deficiency:
cry involuntarily
lack oxygen
anemia
blood lack color
decreased energy
weakness
dizziness
shortness of breath
arthritis
pounding heart
slow mental reactions
pallor
digestive disturbances
fragile bones
nervousness

obesity
dull hearing
sleepless at night
hair loss
brittle hair
pain in heels
palpitations
fatigue
lacking vitality
Alzheimer's
forgetfulness
difficulty swallowing
brittle fingernails with longitudinal ridging, colorlessness
muscle weakness
susceptibility to infection

Nutrients Which Augment:
Vitamins B6
Vitamin B12,
Vitamin C
Folic acid
Copper
Cobalt
Phosphorus
Calcium

Foods & Sources:

pumpkin	blue cohosh root
green leafy vegetables	dates
dried fruits	mullein leaf
alfalfa	chickweed
sea vegetation	avocados
beans	whole grains
seeds	almonds
wheat germ	beets
small amount in all foods	pears
althea root	watercress
bilberry fruit	butchers broom

catnip herb
bayberry bark
dulse
kelp
peaches
devils claw

burdock root
red raspberry leaf
thyme leaf
uva ursi leaf
mullein leaf

Useful For:
aids blood cells
development of tissue respiration
oxygen carrying ability
alcoholism
anemia
colitis
menstrual periods
pregnancy
lactation
Iron function & deficiency anemia
heart
muscle weakness
immune system
obesity
recycles except during menstruation or hemorrhage
not absorbed without hydrocholin, or when taking alkalizing preparations
destroys Vitamin E - take 8 hours apart

MAGNESIUM
Daily Dose - RDA - 300-350 mg
Approx. restore - 300-1,000 mg
Best source - Gluconate or citrate
(adult doses listed; child's dose 9-14 years - 1/2 dose, 2-8 years - 1/3 dose)

Destroyed By:
cortisone
antibiotics
cooked nuts

white bread
milk
sugar
stress
alcohol
diuretics
perspiration
x-ray

Parts of the Body Essential For:
preserving mineral balance
utilization of calcium
acid alkaline balance
blood sugar balance
metabolism of Vitamin C
metabolism of glucose

Symptoms of Deficiency:
confusion
disorientation
anger
irritability
nervousness
rapid pulse
tremors
bed wetting
fear
gas
insomnia
Chronic Fatigue Syndrome
prostate problems
suicidal tendency
irritable bowel syndrome
Epstein-Barr
often synonymous with diabetes
hyperactivity
convulsions
colitis

depression
kidney stone
diarrhea
dizziness
seizures
poor digestion
mental disorder
cardiovascular problem
anxiety
palpitations of heart
yellowish whites in eyes
muscle spasms, twitching
sensitive to noise
herpes
candida
twitching
PMS
muscle aches, pain & weakness
senility
edema
tantrums
asthma

Nutrients Which Augment:
Vitamins B6
Vitamin C
Vitamin D
Calcium
Phosphorus
Potassium
Foods & Sources:

leaf lettuce	lentils
tomatoes	mushrooms
watercress	mustard greens
corn	avocados
leeks	apples
parsnips	apricots
alfalfa chlorophyll	grapefruit

onions
astragalus root
boneset herb
potatoes
peas
spinach
sauerkraut
turnips
garlic
lemons
tofu
peaches
nettle leaf
oat grass straw
nuts
whole grains:
barley
small amount in most foods

rye
wheat
dairy products
burdock root
chickweed
devils claw
elecampane root
horseradish root
kelp
senna leaf
Siberian ginseng root
turmeric herb
white willow bark
yerba santa leaf
dulse
licorice
peppermint leaf

Useful For:
alcoholism
high cholesterol
depression
kidney stones
prostate troubles
stomach acidity
tooth decay
brain
high blood pressure
calcium utilization
endometriosis
glands
Spinal fluid
Alzheimer's
PMS
endometriosis
Chronic Fatigue Syndrome
Epstein Barr

blood vessels
overweight
healthy nervous system
proper body ph balance
heart

When the pituitary is not getting necessary magnesium, it fails in its regulatory function for the adrenal, allowing them to over produce, resulting in anxiety and seeming nervousness.

When the adrenal gland become exhausted from overproduction of adrenal hormones, low blood sugar and inability to cope with stress are the results.

Milk depletes magnesium because the synthetic Vitamin D found in milk binds magnesium. Children who have epilepsy or tendency to convulsions only increase the risk by drinking milk.

Magnesium is necessary in high altitudes to lessen the effort of the heart which must work harder because the small vessels of the lungs tend to constrict in high altitudes. Magnesium makes a change in the process of such constriction.

Processed food could be the cause of exhausted people with so many nervous afflictions and with distorted thinking, because magnesium is destroyed in the processing of foods.

MANGANESE (Trace Mineral) Antioxidant
Daily Dose - RDA - 5 mg
Approx. restore - 10 mg

(adult doses listed; child's dose 9-14 years - 1/2 dose, 2-8 years - 1/3 dose)

Destroyed By:
Choline
Calcium (excessive)
Phosphorus (excessive)

Biotin

Parts of the Body Essential For:
activation of enzymes
reproduction & growth
hormone production
tissue repair
Vitamins B1 & E utilization
important in growth, pregnancy & lactation
proper brain function
muscles
nerves

Symptoms of Deficiency:
multiple sclerosis
muscle coordination failure
dizziness
ear noise
loss of hearing
changes in hair color
tendency to breast ailments
profuse perspiration
atherosclerosis
tooth grinding
memory loss
convulsions
eye problems
pancreatic damage
heart disorders
rapid pulse
confusion
dermatitis

Nutrients Which Augment:
B Complex
For the utilization of B1
Vitamin E

Foods & Sources:

avocados
nuts
brazil nuts
almonds
seeds
seaweed
celery
green leafy vegetables
swiss cheese
turnips
hydrangea root
ginger root
hibiscus root
gotu kola leaf
horseradish root
yellow dock root
whole grains

raspberries
bran
corn
chickweed
devils claw
bilberry fruit
blue cohosh
catnip herb
barley
pineapple
blueberries
legumes
dried peas
beet root
kale
beans
bananas

Useful For:

allergies
asthma
diabetes
fatigue
multiple sclerosis
growth
reproduction
bones
teeth
central nervous system
schizophrenia
osteoarthritis
healthy nerves
fat metabolism
healthy immune system
blood sugar system regulation
cartilage
aids in formation of mother's milk

PHOSPHORUS
Daily Dose - RDA - 800 mg
Approx. restore- 800-1,000 mg
(adult doses listed; child's dose 9-14 years - 1/ 2 dose, 2-8 years - 1/3 dose)

Destroyed By:
antacids
aluminum
iron
magnesium (excessive)
white sugar (excessive)

Parts of the Body Essential For:
bone & teeth formation
cell growth & repair
energy
heart muscles contraction
kidney function
metabolism of calcium and sugar
nerve & muscles activity
vitamin utilization, especially B
nursing mothers
development of cells
metabolism of fats
necessary for mental power

Symptoms of Deficiency:

afraid of tomorrow
dislike of sex, work
fearful
general weakness
loss of muscle tone
numbness of limbs
prone to arthritis
paralysis

anxiety
bone pain
irregular breathing
Alzheimer's
poor growth of hair
skin sensitivity
trembling
tooth decay
Weight Changes:
   weight gain
   weight loss
poor growth of fingernails
irritability
appetite loss
fatigue

Nutrients Which Augment:
Vitamins A, D, F, B6
Calcium
Iron
Manganese
Sodium

Foods & Sources:

dried fruits	broccoli
legumes	buchu
seeds:	cabbage
pumpkin	cauliflower
sunflower	bran
sesame	brewers yeast
nuts	corn
asparagus root	cranberries
bilberry fruit	garlic
blue cohosh root	peppermint leaf
yellow dock root	Siberian ginseng root
hydrangea root	saw palmetto root
yerba santa root	salmon
asparagus	small amounts in all foods

Useful For:
arthritis
stress
endometriosis
tooth & gum disorders
retarded growth in children

Phosphorus is not properly absorbed without sufficient hydrochloric acid in the stomach. With adrenal insufficiency or low blood sugar, phosphorus may not be used by the body. (see "Is Any Sick Among You?" for information on hormone herbs.)

Carbonate soft drinks - high in phosphorous - upsetting the balance of calcium/magnesium

POTASSIUM
Daily Dose - RDA - None
Approx. restore - 3,000-10,000 mg
Best source - gluconate
(adult doses listed; child's dose 9-14 years - 1/2 dose, 2-8 years - 1/3 dose)

Destroyed By:
too much sodium
alcohol
coffee
cortisone
too many laxatives
excessive sugar
stress
salt
diuretics
drug hormones

Parts of the Body Essential For:
alkalinity of body fluids
normal heartbeat
body growth

nerve tranquilization
proper function of digestion

Symptoms of Deficiency:
hypoglycemia
acne
continuous thirst
dry skin
constipation
general weakness
insomnia
muscle damage
nervousness
slow, irregular heartbeats
weak reflexes
water retention
weak ligaments
listlessness
soft, flabby muscles
salt retention
nausea/vomiting
low blood pressure
high cholesterol
growth impairment
swollen testicles or ovaries
chills
depression
diarrhea
edema
Guinne Barré
Epstein-Barr
Chronic Fatigue Syndrome
glucose intolerance
respiratory disease

Nutrients Which Augment:
Vitamin B6
Sodium

Magnesium

Foods & Sources:
dried apricots, 1 C = 1,450 mg
bananas, 1 med = 500 mg
sunflower-seed, 1 C = 900 mg
celery
gooseberries
cucumber
kale
lettuce
cooked onions
sweet potatoes
pumpkin
radishes
rutabaga
squash
brazil nuts
molasses
broccoli
carrots
cabbage
cauliflower
chard
tomatoes
watercress
rice
alfalfa chlorophyl
hickory nuts
barley
eggplant
endive
lentils
leeks
mushrooms
mustard greens

avocados
chestnuts
dates
figs
peaches
prunes
apples
pineapples
strawberries
blueberries
cherries
apricots
cranberries
watermelon
limes
turnip tops and roots
onions
parsley
parsnips
peas
walnuts
sauerkraut
spinach
asparagus
catnip herb
blessed thistle herb
parsley herb
corn
rye

Useful For:

acne
allergies
diabetes
alcoholism
colic
high blood pressure

Leakage of potassium from cells or loss of potassium could be the cause of muscular dystrophy, as potassium is necessary for muscle strength.

Losses Occur By:
spilling off in urine
excessive sodium intake
diuretics (water pills)
ACTH
cortisone
aspirin
alcohol
drinking excessive water
vomiting
stress
diarrhea
drugs

Excessive sugar causes stress, spilling off potassium. This could be more the cause of heart attack than too many fatty acids. Sugar decreases cell potassium, rendering heart and all muscles weak and flabby.

Another reason for heart weakness is the use of too much salt. If the intake is no more than 1 tsp. daily, at least 5,000 mg is required. We Americans consume at least 1 to 5 tsp. of salt daily and do not eat enough fruits and vegetables to make up for the potassium deficiency.

Potassium has been noticeably lacking in leukemia and polio patients. Diabetics lose potassium when high sugar is ingested, causing a potassium deficiency.

SILICON (Trace Mineral)
Daily Dose - RDA- unknown
Approx. restore - unknown

Destroyed By:
Not known

Parts of the Body Essential For:
natural alkalizer
regulate cell tissue

Symptoms of Deficiency:
itchy ears
sties on eyes
ear discharge
ulceration of tongue
sensitive teeth
boils
nervous exhaustion
listlessness
no ambition for brain work

Foods & Sources:
apricots
cherries
endive
cauliflower
asparagus
lima beans
parsley
persimmons
bell peppers
soy beans
green leafy vegetables
horsetail
astragalus root
burdock root
butchers broom root

chickweed
oat grass straw
thyme leaf
dulse
pumpkin
horseradish
lettuce
oranges
olives
almonds
coconut
current
beets
whole grains:
    brown rice

Echinacea root
ginger root
golden seal root
hydrangea root

licorice
horsetail herb
grapevine herb

Useful For:
drug addiction
prevention of Alzheimer's
arteriosclerosis
healthy nails, skin and hair
arthritis
osteoporosis
stimulates immune system

SODIUM (Trace Mineral)
Daily Dose - RDA - 3,000-7,000 mg
Approx. restore - 3,000-10,000 mg
Best Source - celery
(adult doses listed; child's dose 9-14 years - 1/2 dose, 2-8 years - 1/3 dose)

There is a big difference in sodium as it occurs naturally in food, than sodium chloride or table salt.

Destroyed By:
chlorine
lack of potassium

Parts of the Body Essential For:
normal cellular fluid
muscle contraction

Symptoms of Deficiency:
appetite loss
indigestion
muscle shrinkage
intestinal gas
vomiting

weight loss
low blood pressure
hair falling out
loss of sense of smell
early morning exhaustion
heat stroke when in sun too long
heat stroke symptoms:
  nausea, dizziness, vomiting, cramping of leg, back, or abdominal being used at the time

Nutrients Which Augment:
Vitamin D
Potassium
Iron
Phosphorous

Foods & Sources:

grapes
olives
pears
brazil nuts
peanuts
walnuts
herring
prunes
strawberries
watermelon
chestnuts
coconut
swiss cheese
asparagus
beans
Limburger cheese
raw goat milk
molasses
alfalfa
kale
leeks

rutabaga
sauerkraut
okra
squash
turnips
barley eggs
pomegranate
blueberries
cherries
cranberries
dates
gooseberries
dill
carrots
cauliflower
gotu kola leaf
rice
wheat
apples
watercress
corn

egg yolks
avocado
bananas
pineapple
chard
endive
lettuce
celery
beets
parsley herb
carrot

Irish moss
oat grass straw
licorice
parsley
peas
potatoes
rhubarb
tomatoes
limes
lemons

Useful For:
dehydration
fever
heat stroke
natural alkalizer
regulating cell tissues
Alzheimer's disease
healthy skin and hair
Calcium absorption
Counteracts the effect of aluminum in the body
Stimulates the immune system

SULPHUR (Trace Mineral)
Daily Dose - RDA - none
Approx. restore - trace
Best Source - garlic

Destroyed By:
Moisture and heat may destroy or change the action of
sulphur in the body

Parts of the Body Essential For:
body tissue formation
toning blood
improving looks
stimulating liver secretions

called beautifying mineral
needed for synthesis of collagen

Symptoms of Deficiency:
toxic condition
disc trouble
hair dull
joint troubles
voice box gives out easily
joyless appearance
menstruation:
delayed
irregular
sores do not heal
difficulty talking or singing
moodiness

Nutrients Which Augment:
Vitamin B1
B Complex
Biotin
Pantothenic acid

Sulphur of the type not occurring naturally in food is poison to the body. This type is used to sulfur fruits to preserve color.

Foods & Sources:

nuts	whole wheat
wheat germ	corn
raw goat milk	rice
asparagus	bananas
carrots	dates
cauliflower	figs
endive	olives
lettuce	lentils
parsnips	mushrooms
potatoes	mustard greens
peaches	cooked onions

parsley
peas
peppers
sweet potatoes
raisins
pumpkin
radishes
rhubarb
rutabaga
sauerkraut
tomatoes
turnips
watercress
barley
wheat germ
apricots
broccoli
celery
chard
gooseberries
raspberries

grapefruit
grapes
walnuts
blueberries
oranges
watermelon
hickory nuts
molasses
soybeans
lima beans
beets
lemons
limes
coconut
filberts
pecans
eggplant
blackberries
cantaloupe
cherries
cranberries

Useful For:
arthritis
external skin disorders
muscles
brain
skin
bones
helps the body resist bacteria
disinfects the blood
protects the protoplasm of cells
protects against toxic substances

ZINC
Daily Dose - RDA - 50 mg
Approx. restore - 50-100 mg

(adult doses listed; child's dose 9-14 years - 1/2 dose, 2-8 years - 1/3 dose)

Destroyed By:
alcohol
Calcium (high intake)
lack of phosphorus
diarrhea
kidney diseases
liver disease
diabetes
perspiration
hard water
iron (take at different time)

Parts of the Body Essential For:
burns & wound healing
carbohydrate digestion
prostate gland function
reproductive organ growth & development
sex organ growth & development
Vitamin B, phosphorous & protein metabolism

Symptoms of Deficiency:
delayed sexual maturity
fatigue
loss of taste
poor appetite
slow healing of wounds
retarded growth
sterility
prostrate trouble
acne
recurrent colds & flu
hair loss
impaired night vision
impotence
infertility

memory impairment
propensity to diabetes
susceptibility to infection

Nutrients Which Augment:
Vitamins A, B6, E
Calcium
Copper
Phosphorus

Foods & Sources:

brewer's yeast	bran
soybeans	wheat germ
spinach	onions
sunflower seeds	maple syrup
mushrooms	green leafy vegetables
astragalus root	ginkgo biloba leaf
bilberry	elecampane root
capsicum root	saw palmetto root
damiana root	scullcap herb
Echinacea root	Siberian ginseng root
buchu	spirulina algae
dulse	grapevine herb

Useful For:
alcoholism
arteriosclerosis
cirrhosis
diabetes
wounds
high cholesterol
infertility

DNA molecules are the principles of all life forms on earth. When anything is alive it has DNA molecules. This is the characteristic which makes it possible to for new cells and growth.

DNA gives instruction and RNA or ribonucleic acid, does the work, or carries out the genetic plan. Zinc is necessary for DNA to function properly.

Do not take more than 100 mg daily. Up to 100 mg will enhance the immune system while more than 100 mg will depress the immune system.

OTHER TRACE MINERALS

ALUMINUM

Foods & Sources:
althea root
blue cohosh root
butchers broom root
chickweed
echinacea root
ginger root
mullein leaf
thyme leaf
uva ursi leaf
buchu

SELENIUM

Foods & Sources:
althea root
bayberry bark
black cohosh root
black walnut fruit & rind
blessed thistle herb
blue cohosh
catnip herb
milk thistle leaf
buchu
dulse
lemon grass

All herbs have many vitamins and minerals. Those listed are the herbs highest in the particular mineral or vitamin noted here according to the latest studies.

VITAMIN & MINERAL DEFICIENCIES & DISEASES
(To be used in addition to a full vitamin/mineral complex)

ACNE
Vitamin A
Niacin
Potassium
Sulphur
Vitamin B2
Vitamin E

ALCOHOLISM
Pangamic acid
Folic acid
B Complex
Potassium
Zinc
Choline

ALLERGIES
Pantothenic acid
B Complex
Potassium
Manganese
Vitamin F

ALZHEIMER'S DISEASE
B Complex
Niacin
Calcium
Iron
Magnesium
Silicon

Sodium

ANEMIA
Folic acid
B Complex
Vitamin B1
Iron
Copper
Vitamin E
Phosphorus

ANTIOXIDANTS
Vitamin A
Vitamin E
Vitamin C

ANXIETY
Inositol
Pantothenic Acid
Magnesium
Phosphorus

APPETITE LOSS
Zinc
Biotin

ARTERIOSCLEROSIS
Vitamin A
Choline

ARTHRITIS
Pantothenic acid
B Complex
Phosphorus
Sulphur
Calcium
Vitamin F
Vitamin E

ASPIRIN POISONING
Vitamin C

ASTHMA
Vitamin C
Vitamin F
Vitamin P
B Complex
Manganese

ATHEROSCLEROSIS
Iodine
Pangamic acid
Inositol
Folic acid
Zinc
Vitamin B6
Choline
Vitamin F
Biotin

BALDNESS
PABA
Pantothenic acid
Niacin
Inositol
Folic acid
B Complex
Vitamin B6
Biotin
Copper
Vitamin F

BARBITURATE OVERDOSE
B Complex

BLACK WIDOW SPIDER BITES

Vitamin C

BLEEDING GUMS
Vitamin P
Vitamin C

BLOOD CLOTS
Vitamin E

BROKEN BONES
Vitamin E
Calcium
Vitamin C

BRUISES
Vitamin C
Vitamin K

BURNS
Vitamin C
Zinc
PABA
Vitamin E

CANDIDA
Vitamin A
B Complex
Vitamin E

CARBON MONOXIDE POISONING
Vitamin C

CATARACTS
Niacin
Vitamin B2

CHOLESTEROL (ELEVATED)
B Complex

Inositol
Pangamic Acid
Vitamin C
Vitamin D
Vitamin P
Choline
Chromium
Potassium
Zinc

CHRONIC FATIGUE SYNDROME
B Complex
Vitamin B-12
Vitamin C
Vitamin E
Calcium
Magnesium
Potassium

CIRRHOSIS
Zinc

COLD HAND & FEET
Iodine

COLDS
Vitamin C
Pantothenic acid
Vitamin P

COLITIS
Iron
Vitamin E

CONSTIPATION
Choline

CYSTITIS

Pantothenic acid
B Complex

DANDRUFF
Vitamin A

DEHYDRATION
Sodium

DEPRESSION
Biotin
Magnesium

DERMATITIS
Biotin

DETACHED RETINA
Vitamin A

DIABETES
Potassium
Zinc
Manganese
Chromatin

DIARRHEA
Folic acid

DIGESTIVE DISORDERS
Pantothenic acid
Vitamin B2

DISC TROUBLES
Sulphur
Calcium

DIZZINESS
Choline

Manganese
Iron
Vitamin P

DRY SKIN
PABA

ECZEMA
Vitamin B6
Biotin
Vitamin P

EMPHYSEMA
Pangamic acid

ENCEPHALITIS
Vitamin C

EPSTEIN-BARR
B Complex
Vitamin B-12
Vitamin C
Vitamin E
Calcium
Magnesium
Potassium

FATIGUE
Folic acid
Zinc
Manganese
Iron

FEVER
Sodium

FROSTBITE
Vitamin E

GALLSTONES
Vitamin A
Vitamin E

GOITER
Iodine

GRAY HAIR
PABA

GUINNE BARRÉ
Vitamin A
B Complex
Vitamin B-6
Vitamin E
Calcium
Potassium

HAIR COLOR RESTORED
PABA

HAIR LOSS
B Complex
Vitamin A
Vitamin B-2
Vitamin F
Biotin
Folic Acid
Inositol
Iron
Niacin
Pantothenic Acid
Copper
Sodium

HALITOSIS
Niacin

HAY FEVER
Vitamin C

HEADACHE
Choline
Pangamic acid

HEART DISEASE
Pangamic acid
Inositol
Magnesium
Vitamin E

HEATSTROKE
Sodium

HEMORRHAGE
Vitamin K

HEMORRHOIDS
Vitamin B-6
Vitamin P

HERNIA
Vitamin E

HIGH BLOOD PRESSURE
Vitamin C
Vitamin E
Vitamin P
Choline
Calcium
Phosphorus
Potassium
Magnesium

IMMUNE SYSTEM

Vitamin A
Vitamin C
Vitamin E
Folic Acid
Iron
Calcium
Manganese
Sodium

INSOMNIA
Pangamic acid
Choline
Iron
Calcium

JOINT TROUBLES
Sulphur

KIDNEY INFECTION
Vitamin C

KIDNEY STONES
Magnesium
Vitamin C

LEG CRAMPS
Niacin
Biotin
Calcium

LIVER PROBLEMS
Vitamin A

LOSS OF TASTE
Zinc

MENINGITIS
Vitamin C

MENOPAUSE
Calcium

MENSTRUAL CRAMPS
Calcium
Vitamin E

MENSTRUAL PROBLEMS
B Complex
Iron
Vitamin K

MENTAL ILLNESS
Folic acid

MENTAL RETARDATION
Vitamin B6

MIGRAINE HEADACHES
Niacin
Vitamin B Complex

MISCARRIAGE
Vitamin P
Vitamin E

MOTION SICKNESS
Vitamin B6

MOUTH SORES
Vitamin B2
Pantothenic acid
Vitamin B6

MUSCULAR DISORDERS
Vitamin B6
Manganese

NAUSEA
Vitamin B1

NERVOUSNESS
Vitamin B6
Iodine

NEURALGIA
Vitamin B1

NIGHT VISION
Vitamin A

OSTEOPOROSIS
Vitamin D
Chromium
Silicon

OVERACTIVE THYROID
Iodine
Vitamin E
PABA

OVERWEIGHT
Inositol
B Complex
Vitamin B6
Magnesium
Iodine
Calcium
Vitamin F

PAIN
Vitamin B1

PARASITIC DISEASE
PABA

PARKINSON'S DISEASE
Choline
Calcium
Vitamin E
B complex

PHLEBITIS
Vitamin C

POISON OAK OR IVY
Vitamin C

POISONOUS BITES
Vitamin C

POLIO
Vitamin C

POOR CIRCULATION
Pangamic acid

PREMATURE AGING
Pangamic acid
Calcium
PRE-MENSTRUAL SYNDROME (PMS)
Vitamin B-6
Vitamin E
Magnesium

PROSTRATE TROUBLES
Zinc
Magnesium

PSORIASIS
Vitamin F

PSYCHOSIS

B Complex

RADIATION POISON
Vitamin C

RESPIRATORY FLU
Vitamin C
Pantothenic acid

RETARDED GROWTH
Phosphorus
Zinc

RHEUMATIC FEVER
PABA
Vitamin P

RHEUMATISM
Pangamic acid
Vitamin P
Vitamin E
Calcium

ROCKY MTN. SPOTTED FEVER
PABA

SCIATICA
Vitamin B
SENILITY
Niacin

SENSITIVITY TO LIGHT OR SUN
Vitamin B

SHORTNESS OF BREATH
Pangamic acid
Iron

SINUSITIS
Vitamin C
Pantothenic acid
Vitamin E

SKIN SPOTS
PABA

SLIGHT PARALYSIS
Vitamin B

SORE THROAT, STREP
Vitamin C

STERILITY
Zinc
PABA

STOMACH ULCERS
Folic acid
Vitamin P

STRESS
Vitamin C
PABA
Pantothenic acid
Folic acid
B Complex
Phosphorus
Vitamin B6

SUNBURN
PABA

SWOLLEN GLANDS
Vitamin C

TOOTH DECAY

Pantothenic acid
Niacin
Phosphorus
Magnesium
Calcium

ULCERS
Vitamin P
Vitamin E

VIRUS DISEASES
Vitamin C

VOICE BOX GIVES OUT EASILY
Sulphur

WRINKLES
Vitamin A
Vitamin E

CHAPTER 9

MOTHER AND FATHER'S ROLE IN THE HOME
WHERE LOVE IS HEART TO HEART

Society is developing to a point where children are not being taught true and correct principles. Probably because parents have less time, with both parents working. A set of values has been promoted to raise money for things, therefore raising money, not children.

With the baby sitter, called television, violence values are taught, selfishness, greed, and instant gratification. Gun violence takes a child's life every three hours. Every nine minutes a child is arrested on a drug offense. Every minute of every day, an American teenage girl has a baby out of wedlock. Every twenty six seconds, an American child runs away from home. Suicide is the third leading cause of death among young people. Depression is so common among young people. It involves sixteen percent of the males and nineteen percent of the females.

Twenty percent of all American children are living below poverty level, but most have a television and can see all the things they can wish for. Two and a half million children in the US do not have a permanent home.

The national high school dropout rate is twenty five percent. National average SAT scores have dropped seventy percent in the last thirty years.

Twenty five percent of American girls and thirty three percent of boys, have sexual intercourse by the age of fifteen. Ten thousand babies a year are born to girls less than fifteen years of age. Junior and senior high school students drink thirty five percent of all wine coolers sold in the United States. Forty-one point two (41.2), report use of tobacco in some form.

More than five percent of school children own a gun. Three point six million high school students are assaulted annually. More teenage boys die of gunshot wounds than all other causes combined.

On the television, ten channels, including the three major networks, according to a report in 1992, showed one thousand eight hundred and forty-six individual acts of violence resulting in fatalities. Three hundred eighty nine serious assaults, and three hundred sixty-two using gun play, six hundred and seventy-three scenes using punching, slapping, or pushing.

What kind of a life can children today hope for?

My youngest son asked me to write in this book how to raise children as well as how to feed them. This chapter is simply a mother's opinion.

I have noticed in church the people who give talks about how to raise children usually have only little tiny children. When the children grow up, everyone decides they really did not know anything about how to raise children.

In my field, I have become an expert and I know what I know to be true and if anyone chooses to live by the things I teach about diet, I know they will be blessed physically, spiritually, mentally, socially, and financially.

When your children are grown up and gone from home, there is always the tug at the heart strings. Did I do enough? Did I say enough? Did I say too much? Could I have spent more time with them? Was I a good enough example? Did I love them enough? Did I give them enough? Did I give them too much?

My written books and lectures really began with my family as I learned all these things and applied them to our lives, but I did not begin to write and lecture until my family was almost raised. My youngest son Scott has traveled many miles with me. By age seventeen, he had logged more air miles than most people ever see in a lifetime.

What I did with my children in a health way paid off, and they were all beautiful healthy children. As I watch them now with their own little families, some of them have not followed our way and some of them have. All I can say is I did the best I could with the knowledge I had and what I did for them was all done with love in mind. It was full all the way. The happiest times of my life were when we were raising our family.

Everyone has their own way and free agency, and all I can say is what we did. I know it worked for us.

What I wanted were good, well-behaved children, a clean house, a peaceful home where there was no quarreling and no meanness, a house of love and prayer, a place of refuge from the world. A place of learning. A place for everyone to come home where there was reflected the sweet spirit of the Lord. I wanted the children to be obedient and kind to each other and to us. For the most part that is what we have had.

The only way I can say that it was achieved is this: we tried to follow the guide lines of a religious life. We love the children and each other. We seldom had a baby sitter. We took the children everywhere with us. We simply enjoyed each other. We never allowed the children to quarrel or hit each other.

The way I disciplined the children (the job of discipline became mine, because I was the one at home) was to be consistent. I remember a friend of mine saying "You should put everything up to adult eye level while the children are growing up and have decent things when the children are grown." I did not believe that; at least it wasn't right for me. We surrounded the children with beauty and taught them to take care of it.

Most of our children are artists and musicians; creative people. They needed beauty and art, music and the love that went with an ascetic type person.

It all goes back to deciding what you want, not just for your children, but for yourself as well.

If parents are going to teach children in a certain way, they must be consistent. If you threaten them, you must be ready to follow through. If you promise, you must keep your word. It doesn't require spanking and yelling at children to make them obedient; it requires mother (or whoever is in charge of discipline) to always be on top of the situation, always responding consistently. Then the child knows who you are and what you expect. It's like keeping a schedule. The children always know they can count on you to do and say what you do.

If a child refused to comply with the rules there was punishment, usually grounding, but we always tried to be polite to our children, letting them save face, so they have been polite with us. We did not swear at them, so they didn't ever swear at us. We have always tried to make our home peaceful. We taught them all the positive virtues and tried always to build their self esteem.

It all goes back to what you want, and we worked hard at what we wanted. What we wanted and what our grown children will want maybe entirely different. I know people who are stimulated by a good old knockdown, drag out fight and think it would be so fun to make up. When I watch some married couples and how rudely they talk to each other, I wonder how they stay together. I would be devastated by that kind of treatment. All in all, I think our children have grown up to be responsible people, honest and fair in their dealings and likeable. What kind of home they make will be their choice, but we had the kind we wanted and it was a happy and loving home.

Children understand their parents very fast and they learn what to expect. If the parents are consistent in certain things, the children respond in kind. If there is fighting, quarreling, nagging, harassing, blaming, antagonism, or abuse, the children will respond. They will grow to love you or hate you for whatever you consistently are.

It is a frightening thing when God gives you a tiny baby when you are eighteen years old like I was with my first baby. What did I know about babies or raising kids? I was only a dumb kid myself, but I knew what I wanted my home to be, and I have worked hard to make it so.

Here are some of the main things I tried to teach my children aside from walking and talking. Not listed in order of importance, but rather the things I felt I wanted to teach them. How well I succeeded remains to be seen.

Teach them to love; forgetting self.
Teach them not to quarrel; turn the other cheek, be a peacemaker, walk away from a fight.
Teach them to be kind and Christ like.
Teach them the Gospel of Jesus Christ; stories and principles.
Teach them the value of time and to recognize priorities.
Teach them that time is a most valuable commodity.
Teach them life is short but eternity is forever.
Teach them to be honorable, just and honest.
Teach them to make judgments about whom they will associate with; that it is not their right to judge anyone's punishment for wrong doings.
Teach them to conserve and take care of what they have.
Teach them to learn and how to learn.
Teach them the Lord's Commandments and teach them to obey what the Lord had commanded.
Teach them how to finish what they start.
Teach them to be responsible for their own actions.

Teach them how to serve others.

Teach them to be honest with themselves and others.

Teach them to forgive themselves and others.

Teach them to be morally clean.

Teach them about the atonement of Christ and the principle of repentance.

Teach them to obey the laws of the land as well as the laws of the Lord.

Teach them to pray and have faith in the Lord's answering their prayers.

Teach them to appreciate the beauty of the world.

Teach them to love and enjoy beauty in all of life.

Teach them that wickedness never was happiness, that real happiness and joy are only found in righteous living, surrounded with the light of Christ.

Teach them to work.

Teach them to be clean and orderly.

Teach them to eat right to stay well.

Teach them the cause of illness and how to heal the body.

Teach them to be independent.

I am thankful for the experience with all of my children. They have probably taught me as much as I have taught them, and it has been wonderful. I have had a wonderful husband and we have shared a good life together. If I can give any advice at all, it would be to say you get what you want; just make up your mind, then work hard for it. Love, and give a lot.

What people talk about? :

1: The shallow person talks about people and sees only
what others do? Criticism or gossip or even lies are their main topic of conversation.

2: The mediocre person talks about things. Houses,
furniture, cars, money, and possessions are important to them. They collect things to show off. They compete with others to see who

can accumulate the most things. These things fill the topics of their conversations.

3: The caring person talks about ideas. How to improve the world and make it better. They are fascinated with the idea of making everything better from building, to electronics. Their conversations are all about improvement for the betterment of mankind.

4: The scientist talks about things that few people understand. He or she lives in a world of questions, and for the most part lives alone with thought and reason. This type needs to know everything. They dig and pry and study endlessly to find one small answer. They must know how it all works, from the smallest matter to the largest universe. Their conversation is filled with everything from the questions to the latest discovery of a truth.

5: The spiritual person lives in the spirit and seeks to learn everything and be led alone by the spirit to answers. They expect answers to their questions or their problems and patiently waits for answers or miracles, whichever is asked for. The more spiritual this type becomes, the more they have a desire to help their fellow men to find the faith, love, and peace, they have found. If they have developed an unconditional love, no one is excluded from their help wealthy, or poor, weak, or strong, sick, or well. Their conversation is in a realm which lifts, and helps, never hurts or sees the weakness of others or their shame, only showing love, tenderness, and help.

In conclusion the following statement must be made if anyone even the most sickly are to receive benefit from this book. They must begin to realize that they cannot eat the same as the person who has a strong inherent body. Anyone who is born with chronically inherent disease automatically proceeds to deteriorate in their condition, if they eat an ordinary diet. A mother with a sickly weak child who recognizes this early could save her child's life and bless the child's life beyond measure.

A person who was born with a strong healthy body seems to be able to disobey all the rules of health. This person knowingly or unknowingly even fully aware may break all the rules of health and seem to go unpunished. Much like the eighty-year-old man who brags that he has smoked and drank liquor most of his life and never had a sick day. He will usually have little empathy for sick people's complaints about their aches and pains. His philosophy is usually "think positive sickness is all in your mind." Because the person born with the wonderfully healthy body, thinks he can always get away with disobedience to the laws of nature, it is a great shock to him when he finally realizes he has beaten his body to death. What a waste.

J. M. Gibby said:
"Death is a gradual process only its consummation seems sudden."

To you mother's, who have unhealthy children, may you discover that as you learn the things I have presented to you, and apply them to your children, it will make a difference in their life as well as yours.

Return to the section on mild food and incorporate it in your lifestyle, testing it thoroughly. And you will find what I have told you is a wonderful truth. When vitamins, minerals and herbs are added to the regiment for a particular problem area health will greatly improve.

As you begin to put these truths into practice, you will find that your family will be blessed as mine has and it will fill you with amazement and gratitude. I have spoken here to the mother's particularly no matter how society and the need to earn a living has changed, the duty of nurturing still falls on the mother. In those rare times when father takes the roll he also needs to learn these truths. If mother neglects her roll during pregnancy or in the early days of her child's life, with the exception of inherent weakness from the family genitors, the fault is hers and she must learn to live with the disobedience to the laws of health, along with her child.

"Good health and a good marriage are fleeting things, requiring a constant vigil and hard consistent effort in order to keep them."

A child that is well nourished in body and mind is a happy child who does not have the hidden hungers that lead to drugs, sex, or foodless foods. They seek out these negative things in order to find peace, energy, or relaxation, all of which can be greatly helped through proper nutrition. When your body feels well from correct eating, life becomes the great adventure that it should be. You think clearer, the ability to reason and learn, is enhanced, there is less anger, less frustration, and more hope for the future. May your children be able to enjoy the wonder and beauty of life to its fullest and may you decide now to choose health for your children.

INDEX

Emphysema - 155, 208
Encephalitis - 49, 15, 208
Enema - 23, 35, 41, 51-55, 57, 65-70, 73, 75, 91
Epilepsy - 139, 184
Epstein-Barr -128, 138, 158, 172, 181, 190, 208
Estrogen - 162
Eyes - 56, 93, 107, 114, 116, 124, 125, 127, 129, 132, 133, 138,
    163, 164, 182, 193

F
Fainting - 135
Fasting - 16, 18, 20, 22, 23, 24, 25, 78, 108, 109
Fatigue - 76, 88, 95, 125-127, 135, 138, 144, 145, 148, 150, 153,
    154, 176, 179, 186. 188, 199, 208
Fenugreek - 130, 133
Fever - 19, 38, 41, 51, 52, 55, 61, 66, 67, 68, 70, 75, 83, 129,
    131, 196, 208
Flu - 18, 53, 152, 168, 197, 215
Folic Acid - 32, 137, 143
Frostbite - 163, 208

G
Gallstones - 125, 165, 209
Gastritis - 150
Garlic - 67, 177, 183, 188, 196
Gas - 25, 30, 107, 138, 152, 181, 194
Gibby, J. M. - 9, 45, 225
Ginger - 41, 55, 186, 194, 201
Ginseng - 183, 188, 200
Glands - 36, 49, 64, 66, 67, 70, 74, 95, 106, 107, 111, 134, 141,
    143, 150, 183,
Glaucoma - 50, 132, 150, 156
Glycerin - 55
Goiter - 176, 177, 209
Golden Seal - 34-36, 52, 56, 57, 67, 68, 70, 75, 88, 91, 112-115,
    194
Gout - 50, 150, 156
Gray Hair - 144, 151, 152, 153, 154, 175, 209

Guinne Barré - 126, 128, 135 158, 1625 172, 190, 209

H

Hair - 35, 39, 105, 124, 127, 129, 140, 141, 166, 172, 175, 177, 185, 188, 194, 196

Hair Dull - 35, 176, 197

Hair Loss - 125, 133, 135, 146, 179, 195, 199, 209

Hallucinations - 138

Hay Fever - 49, 158, 210

Hawthorn Berries - 86

Headache - 19, 68, 128, 135, 138, 143, 148, 149, 150, 152, 155, 210

Healing Crisis - 22, 23, 77

Heart - 52, 76, 81-88, 97, 128-131, 138, 140, 143, 145, 154, 160, 161, 163, 164, 170, 172, 178, 180, 182, 184, 185, 187, 189, 190

Heart Attack- 86, 95, 165, 192

Heart Disease - 84-86, 147, 155, 210

Heat Stroke - 195, 210

Hemorrhage - 103, 114, 144, 155, 167, 180, 210

Hemorrhoids - 135,169,210

Hepatitis - 142, 143, 156, 165

Hernia - 164, 210

High Blood Pressure-31, 58, 85, 87, 142, 149, 158, 163, 165, 169, 183, 192, 210

Honey - 18, 21, 39, 41, 44, 105, 107, 108, 128

Hops - 34, 41, 42, 74, 75, 151

Horsetail - 54, 69, 90, 173, 193, 194

Hyperactivity - 170, 181

Hyperglycemia - 100, 102, 128, 173

Hypoglycemia - 66, 72, 143, 150, 152, 161, 173, 190

Infection - 35, 56, 64, 67, 69, 102, 108, 109, 120, 126, 127, 156 177, 179, 200

Inflammation - 54, 55, 69, 83, 88, 99, 102, 159, 160, 177

Inherent Weakness - 225

Inositol - 142, 146, 164

Insomnia - 125, 127, 132, 140, 143, 144, 147, 148, 155, 161, 171, 181, 190, 211

Insulin - 36, 72, 74, 100-115, 173
Iodine - 55, 98, 176, 177
Irritability - 130, 139, 146, 152, 153, 170, 176, 181, 188
Iron - 27, 97, 113 124, 157, 162, 176, 177, 180, 187, 199
Juniper Berries - 35, 54, 69, 88, 89, 91, 112, 113, 173

K

Kelp - 98, 109, 130, 133, 139, 172, 176, 177, 180, 183
Kidney - 26, 50, 51, 54, 55, 66, 69, 74, 88, 89, 90, 91, 96, 100, 103, 107, 112, 115, 142, 142, 158, 159, 172, 187
Kidney Disease - 88, 199
Kidney Infection - 35, 49, 88, 91, 158, 211
Kidney Stone - 33, 91, 92, 137, 182, 183, 211

L

Lactation - 39, 40, 126, 170, 174, 177, 180, 185
Lactic Acid - 66, 73, 130
Lady Slipper - 55, 74, 75, 82, 83, 86, 98, 99
Laxative - 37, 39, 41, 54, 55, 57, 65, 66, 68, 69, 89, 99, 137, 189
Laxative Herbs - 35, 66, 70, 84, 90
Lecithin - 141, 142, 143, 146
Lemon - 65, 67, 68, 70, 91, 92, 157, 183, 196, 198
Leukemia - 192
Licorice - 36, 74, 77, 79, 80, 82, 84, 98, 99, 183, 194, 196
Liver - 22, 50, 91, 99, 106, 107, 112-114, 125-127, 130, 132, 138, 142, 146, 162, 172, 196, 199, 211
Lobelia - 68, 73-75, 83, 86, 91
Low Blood Pressure - 49, 110, 130, 150, 156, 190, 195
Low Blood Sugar - 36, 72, 95, 102, 103, 105, 109, 131, 148, 156, 173, 181, 184,
Lungs - 73-74
Lymph - 69, 99, 150
Magnesium - 73, 79, 80, 90, 97, 98, 136, 137, 157, 171, 180, 184
Malarial parasite - 77
Mandrake - 83, 84, 98, 99
Manganese - 97, 98, 115, 130, 164, 171, 184, 188, 202
Marshmallow - 73, 82, 83, 90
Measles - 49, 54, 55, 59, 60, 64

Ovaries - 95, 190
Overactive Thyroid - 153, 213
Overweight - 76, 106, 128, 136, 147, 166, 172, 184, 213

P
PABA - 151-154
Pain - 11, 25, 47, 48, 54, 56, 61, 64, 68, 69, 76, 77, 80, 81, 87, 88, 91, 99, 129, 138, 164, 169, 172, 213
Palpitations - 88, 170, 179, 182
Pancreas - 102-106, 111, 113, 134
Pantothenic Acid - 196, 136, 144, 149, 153, 197
Paralysis - 60, 92, 95, 129, 187, 216
Parasites - 19, 24, 25, 63, 65, 77, 79, 84, 106, 109, 110, 111, 116, 122
Parkinson's Disease - 128, 142, 163, 171, 214
Parsley - 42, 91, 98, 99, 113, 126
Peppermint - 34, 67, 125, 183, 188
Phlebitis - 49, 158, 214
Phosphorous - 161, 189, 195, 199
Pimples - 55
Pituitary - 83, 100, 101, 112, 184
Pleurisy - 55
Pneumonia - 23, 39, 40, 53, 55, 64, 108, 125
Poison Oak or Ivy - 214
Poke Root - 66, 82, 84
Polio - 49, 51, 55, 58, 59, 60, 158, 160, 192, 214
Poor Circulation - 105, 130, 155, 214
Potassium - 35, 73, 78-80, 85, 89, 91, 94-98, 100, 115, 134, 189, 192
Pregnancy - 10, 24, 39, 40, 101, 126, 134, 135, 137, 145, 170, 174, 180, 185
Premature Aging - 155, 214
Prostate - 181, 183, 199
Protein - 16, 21, 22, 24-32, 40, 48, 65, 96, 100, 103, 106-109, 112, 124, 127, 132, 134, 137, 140, 142, 144, 152, 154
Psoriasis - 125, 135, 166, 214
Psychosis - 128, 214
Pumpkin Seeds - 111, 115, 154

Puncture Wound - 56, 57
Pyorrhea - 161
Pyridoxine - 134-137

R
Radiation Poisoning - 49, 157, 215

Rash - 55, 77, 148
Raspberry - 42, 98, 99, 113, 151,180
Red Clover - 54, 75, 86, 175
Respiratory Flu - 152, 215
Rheumatism - 119, 135, 155, 169, 215
Rheumatic Fever - 50, 86, 153, 156, 169, 215
Riboflavin - 32, 131, 133
Rocky Mountain Spotted Fever - 154, 215
Rosehips - 66, 157

S
Sage - 42
Sassafras - 35
Scarlet Fever - 86
Senna - 66, 90, 125, 173, 183
Silicon - 99, 193
Sinus - 49, 135, 152
Sinusitis - 135, 157, 158, 164, 216
Skin - 55, 66, 73, 141, 148, 168, 172, 175, 175, 194, 196,
Skin Problems - 77, 88, 89, 104, 115, 124, 127, 135, 136, 153,
    164, 175, 188, 198
Skin Spots - 153, 216
Slippery Elm - 35, 82, 83, 90, 92
Smallpox - 55
Snake Bites - 48, 57
Sodium - 80, 89, 96, 99, 100, 134, 139, 177, 188, 189, 192, 194
Sore Throat, Strep - 49, 55, 64, 68, 95, 157, 161, 216
Sorrel - 115
Spleen - 76, 138, 172
Strawberry - 113
Sulphur - 35, 36, 130, 196, 197

Swollen Glands - 158, 216

T
Teeth - 39, 124, 161, 172, 176, 186, 187
Teeth Problems - 49, 105, 151, 155, 156, 161, 193
Thiamine - 129
Thyme - 173, 180, 193, 201
Thymus - 142, 143
Thyroid - 112, 114, 130, 153, 165
Tonsils - 150
Toxemia - 36, 135
Tumor - 22, 23, 102
Typhoid - 55

U
Ulcer - 50, 51, 126, 143, 150, 156, 160, 166, 169, 193, 217
Ulcer of Stomach - 145, 165, 216

V
Vaginal Problems - 138
Valerian - 74, 75, 86
Varicose Veins - 50, 156, 163, 166, 168
Violet - 125
Virus Diseases - 19, 49, 53, 55, 64, 158, 217
Vitality - 18, 19, 23, 53, 179
Vitamins:
   A - 124-126
   B (complex) - 51, 56, 79, 87, 96, 105, 111, 123, 126-128, 140,
       159
   B_1 (thiamine) - 96, 99, 129, 131, 136, 185
   B_2 (riboflavin) - 32, 130-132, 133, 136, 149
   B_3 (Niacin) - 66, 88, 96, 98, 99, 130, 133, 147, 149
   B_6 (Pyridoxine) - 134-137
   B_{12} (Cobalt) - 137, 174, 175, 179
   B_{15} (Pangamic Acid) -154
   C - 12, 35, 37, 41, 48-52, 54, 55, 57, 66-70, 74, 75, 155-160,
       168, 169, 174, 176
   D - 78-80, 124, 160-162, 184

www.ingramcontent.com/pod-product-compliance
Lightning Source LLC
Chambersburg PA
CBHW060333290526
45793CB00003B/609